Bereavement:
Client Adaptation
and Hospice Services

Bereavement: Client Adaptation and Hospice Services

Donna Lind Infeld, PhD
Nadine Reimer Penner, ACSW, LSCSW
Editors

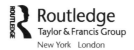

Routledge
Taylor & Francis Group
New York   London

Bereavement: Client Adaptation and Hospice Services has also been published as *The Hospice Journal*, Volume 11, Number 4 1996.

The development, preparation, and publication of this work has been undertaken with great care. However, the publisher, employees, editors, and agents of The Haworth Press and all imprints of The Haworth Press, Inc., including The Haworth Medical Press and Pharmaceutical Products Press, are not responsible for any errors contained herein or for consequences that may ensue from use of materials or information contained in this work. Opinions expressed by the author(s) are not necessarily those of The Haworth Press, Inc.

First published by

The Haworth Press, Inc., 10 Alice Street, Binghamton, NY 13904-1580 USA

This edition published 2012 by Routledge

Routledge
Taylor & Francis Group
711 Third Avenue
New York, NY 10017

Routledge
Taylor & Francis Group
27 Church Road
Hove East Sussex BN3 2FA

Library of Congress Cataloging-in-Publication Data

Bereavement : client adaptation and hospice services/Donna Lind Infeld, Nadine Reimer Penner, editors.
     p. cm.
    Includes bibliographical references and index.
    ISBN 0-7890-0030-X (alk. paper)–ISBN 0-7890-0307-4 (pbk.)
    1. Bereavement–Psychological aspects. 2. Death–Psychological aspects. 3. Grief. 4. Counseling. I. Infeld, Donna Lind. II. Penner, Nadine Reimer.
BF575.G7B45 1996   96-38929
155.9'37–dc21   CIP

Bereavement:
Client Adaptation and Hospice Services

CONTENTS

ABOUT THE EDITORS

Donna Lind Infeld, PhD, is Professor of Health Services Management and Policy and of Health Care Sciences at The George Washington University in Washington, D.C., where she has been on the faculty since 1978. The former Chair of the Association of University Programs in Health Administration Long-Term Care Project Advisory Committees, she has held elected positions in The Gerontological Society of America and is a member of the District of Columbia Board of Examiners for Nursing Home Administrators. Dr. Infeld has published numerous long-term care and hospice research articles and co-edited 3 books. She teaches courses in gerontology and long-term care administration, program evaluation and research methods, health information systems, human behavior, and human resources.

Nadine Reimer Penner, ACSW, LSCSW, is Director of Bereavement and Clinical Social Work for Hospice Incorporated in Wichita, Kansas. Ms. Penner is certified by the American Red Cross as a disaster mental health instructor. The first Bereavement Section Chair of the National Council of Hospice Professionals, she continues to serve on the Bereavement Section Steering Committee. Ms. Penner was appointed by the National Hospice Organization to the National Funeral Director's Association Clergy and Caregivers Committee.

Preface

As a farmer's daughter, I might initially be complimented by the analo-
gy of comparing bereavement counselors to John Deere plows. In my
family, John Deere implements were viewed as the top of the line! Yet
compliments are not what John McKnight in his book *The Careless Society: Community and Its Counterfeits* has in mind.[1]

McKnight, director of Northwestern University's Community Studies
Program for Urban Affairs and Policy Research, tells the story of the
blacksmith, John Deere, who invented a tool sharp enough to plow the
prairie. When the settlers arrived on the prairie by the Wisconsin River,
they brought the plow with them. The plow was used to prepare the sod for
planting wheat. Within thirty years the soil was depleted of its nutrients
even though the Sauk Indians had been able to sustain the prairie for
generations. Many farmers left the area as they could no longer support
themselves off of the land.

According to McKnight, bereavement counseling will have a similar
impact on a community as the John Deere plow. He predicts the demise
of the person's own supportive community. First the bereaved's community would be told the counseling is just to assist the community in
helping the bereaved. Next the local government would be asked to pay
for the counseling of those who could not afford it. Eventually neighbors
would stop dropping by the home of the newly bereaved because they
didn't want to interrupt the bereavement counselor. Within a generation's
time the community surrounding the grieving member would have disap-
peared.

McKnight's words are not easy to swallow. I doubt any of us would say
we are deliberately trying to erode an individual's support system. But is
that what we are subtly doing when we talk about factors predisposing an

[Haworth co-indexing entry note]: "Preface." Penner, Nadine Reimer. Co-published simultaneous-
ly in *The Hospice Journal* (The Haworth Press, Inc.) Vol. 11, No. 4, 1996, pp. 1-3; and: *Bereavement:
Client Adaptation and Hospice Services* (ed: Donna Lind Infeld, and Nadine Reimer Penner) The
Haworth Press, Inc., 1996, pp. 1-3. Single or multiple copies of this article are available for a fee from The
Haworth Document Delivery Service [1-800-342-9678, 9:00 a.m. - 5:00 p.m. (EST). E-mail address:
getinfo@haworth.com].

individual to complicated grief? The National Hospice Organization's bereavement standards require an "assessment of the needs of the bereaved family."[2] The assessment is to include risk factors and the potential for pathological grief reactions. Nowhere does it ask for an assessment of the knowledge, talents, resources and motivations of the bereaved family. What are we saying when we focus on what's wrong without placing at least an equal importance on the strengths of the individual? Dennis Saleebey, Professor, School of Social Welfare, University of Kansas, says "the strengths approach requires an accounting of what people know and what they can do, however inchoate that may sometimes seem. It requires composing a roster of resources existing within and around the individual, family or community."[3]

I am not suggesting communities are always as supportive as they could be or that all individuals have the resources they need to cope with devastating loss. Hospice bereavement programs are dealing with people who have very complex problems as this issue indicates. We need to know how they have dealt with those problems including previous experiences with loss and what they have learned as a result. Then we can begin to help individuals gather their knowledge and resources to deal with their grief and in so doing find strength and hope.

Perhaps Walter Goodman in his review of the Home Box Office documentary "Letting Go: A Hospice Journey" has a valid point when he states many patients and their families are "put off by the prospect of having strangers suddenly involve themselves in one's intimate moments, especially when the newcomers can seem a bit too sure of their perceptions regarding people they really don't know all that well."[4]

Healthy resolution of grief continues to be redefined and the authors in this volume add to our understanding. However, hospice bereavement programs cannot view themselves as the only experts on grief. Rather, they should focus on working collaboratively with the bereaved instead of making assumptions about the correct way to grieve.

Farmers are learning from the Sauk Indians. Many are using the disk rather than the plow and tilling the soil less frequently to preserve the rich nutrients. Hospice bereavement programs must want to learn from bereaved families or else risk taking away the very hope and dignity they seek to give.

Nadine Reimer Penner, ACSW, LSCSW

NOTES

1. John McKnight, *The Careless Society Community and Its Counterfeits* (New York: Basic Books, 1995): 3-15.

2. National Hospice Organization, *Standards of a Hospice Program of Care* (Arlington, Virginia: National Hospice Organization, 1994): 55.

3. Dennis Saleebey, "The Strengths Perspective in Social Work Practice: Extensions and Cautions," *Social Work* (May 1996): 296-305.

4. Walter Goodman, "The Art of Making Life Easier As It Nears An End," *The New York Times* (March 18, 1996).

Saying Hello Again:
A New Approach
to Bereavement Counseling

Shira Ruskay

SUMMARY. It is generally accepted that the successful resolution of grief work is to say goodbye to the deceased. Yet many bereaved resist this therapeutic agenda, reluctant to relinquish the love object. By examining the aspects of the relationship which the bereaved is reluctant to forfeit, grief work can become an opportunity for the bereaved to incorporate the lost relationship into the present and future. The griever is encouraged to say 'hello' again to those aspects that were expressed in the lost relationship thus gaining greater personal integration and wholeness. *[Article copies available for a fee from The Haworth Document Delivery Service: 1-800-342-9678. E-mail address: getinfo@haworth.com]*

Shira Ruskay, MA, JD, CSW, had careers in special education and law before going back to Social Work school to do hospice work. She has been associated with the Visiting Nurse Service of New York Hospice since 1989 as both a clinician and Social Work Coordinator.

Address correspondence to: Shira Ruskay, MA, JD, CSW, 215 West 88th Street, New York, NY 10024.

[Haworth co-indexing entry note]: "Saying Hello Again: A New Approach to Bereavement Counseling." Ruskay, Shira. Co-published simultaneously in *The Hospice Journal* (The Haworth Press, Inc.) Vol. 11, No. 4, 1996, pp. 5-14; and: *Bereavement: Client Adaptation and Hospice Services* (ed: Donna Lind Infeld, and Nadine Reimer Penner) The Haworth Press, Inc., 1996, pp. 5-14. Single or multiple copies of this article are available for a fee from The Haworth Document Delivery Service [1-800-342-9678, 9:00 a.m. - 5:00 p.m. (EST). E-mail address: getinfo@haworth.com].

> The fundamental crisis of bereavement arises,
> not from the loss of other
> but the loss of self.

–Peter Marris

What do we hear when the bereaved broken heart says "When my loved one died, a part of me died too?" If we take this to be only a figure of speech, a way of expressing the enormity of loss or the depth of depression, our inquiry stops here and we respond–appropriately–with empathic nods and noises. But if we enter the world of the metaphor and ask: "What part of you got buried with the bones of your beloved?" the field of inquiry deepens, an auxiliary source of healing emerges, and there is a very real possibility that the successful resolution of grief work will be greater wholeness and integration for the survivor.

THE THEORY

All psychological frameworks endeavor to explain the human experience of being in our essence more than we have access to in daily life, the experience of partiality, of longing for a lost wholeness. There seems to be some basic instinctual nature, some Eden-like state of completeness which is intuited as our natural state. As Robert Bly once said "we come into the world as infants, trailing clouds of glory . . . with a 360° radiance."[1] But in order for the defenseless, dependent newborn to gain the love, approval and protection of family, community, school and society, we increasingly compromise aspects of our fullness, tossing our "unacceptable" parts into a big black bag which we drag along behind us into the sunset.[2] This socialization, this process of disownment, itself produces mourning. Our souls long for the wholeness that has been lost, for the disowned energies that have been socialized into submission but yearn to be expressed.[3] These unexpressed energies and our longing for wholeness accumulate power like water behind a dam. They become the stuff we bring to our chiropractors and to our psychiatrists, the stuff we encounter in our dreams, our fantasies, our sublimations. They become our shadow material, our addictions,[4] our lifelong "if-only"s and deathbed regrets. And these disowned energies or Selves find expression in our relationships.[5]

Through some mysterious, unconscious selection process, we form relationships in which our disowned energies can find expression–sometimes directly but sometimes vicariously, sometimes by being made manifest, sometimes by being affirmatively contained. As a rule of thumb, anyone whom we especially admire or overvalue, and anyone about whom we have especially strong negative feelings, is someone who is expressing a part of *us* that we can't allow ourselves to express. Further, the thing we idolize or despise in the other is the very aspect of ourselves that is forbidden and conflictual.[6]

How is all of this relevant to bereavement? Because we use relationships in part to express our own forbidden Selves, part of what is lost when the beloved dies is the relationship in which that longed-for part of ourselves lived. We grieve not only for the beloved but also for the relationship which made it possible for our own disowned energy to be expressed.[7]

While a first principle of bereavement is that successful resolution of grief is saying goodbye to the beloved, it is also true, as Michael White has suggested,[8] that the problem for the bereaved may be having said goodbye too well to that aspect of the Self that lived in the relationship with the beloved—i.e. in having buried too deep with the bones of the beloved "the part of me that died too." Peter Marris said it so well: "The fundamental crisis of bereavement arises, not from the loss of others, but the loss of self."[9] By bringing that lost aspect of Self to consciousness, the bereaved may reclaim, or say hello again, to parts of her[10] 360° radiance that have been buried.

THE PARADIGMS

Since I first encountered this fertile idea of Michael White's, I have observed in my patients three basic paradigms of how this principle operates in relationships. In the first paradigm, the beloved had facilitated or made it safe for the survivor herself to express a disowned part of her 360° soul. Often there is a cherished aspect of each of us that only one special someone knows about and encourages, a Self that is safely expressed only in that relationship. In this paradigm, the loss of the beloved person is also the loss of this cherished vision of the Self; the loss of the place where it was safe to express the survivor's own forbidden, disowned, private persona.

To illustrate, I shall describe my bereavement work with Delores, a 44-year-old Afro-American nurse at a New York City hospital. When her 46-year-old sister Barbara died of a brain tumor on our hospice program, Delores became the oldest of six siblings. Delores had been at the launching stage in her life cycle when her 47-year-old mother died twenty-two years ago. But having been taught that it's bad to be selfish, and that "it's dangerous out there," Delores tabled her own individuation agenda—indefinitely—and took on the role of family matriarch. Over the years she worked hard to support her daughter and more than one dysfunctional family member, trying, with Barbara's support, to hold together the remnants of the large clan. This onerous status quo had its own compensatory satisfaction while Barbara was alive. The sisters had been closest, dearest friends. They spoke to each other daily, vacationed together, partied together. Barbara was Delores' cheerleader. It was she who could make Delores get herself dressed, kick up her heels, and go out to "do the town."

With Barbara's death, Delores buried her own playfulness and began to feel the full extent and impact of her enormous sacrifice all these years. Several exacerbating features made the situation even more poignant. Delores' daughter was graduating from high school and contemplating whether or not to leave home. She was thus at the very launching stage where Delores had gotten stuck. Delores, with worsening glaucoma and high blood pressure, was approaching the age at which both her mother and Barbara had died. And, as we talked, she revealed a significant bit of family history: One week after Delores' mother's death, another of her mother's sisters died, which so overwhelmed their third sister that she refused to go back to work, becoming functionally disabled by her grief. Delores had inherited a family legacy that says one doesn't always survive the death of a sister.

Delores' work to reclaim, to say hello again to her own disowned playfulness in a Barbara-less world included a lengthy sojourn in deepest anhedonia, pain and despair. But a breakthrough came when, thirteen months after Barbara's death, Delores returned from a long weekend trip to Las Vegas grinning from ear to ear and confessing she hadn't even called home. (Only the second time in her life–the first time she went away and didn't call home, her father had died!) She'd gone with a group of coworkers and had had some risky adventures including flying over a canyon in a "cracker jack box." She'd slept little and lost every penny of the money she had set aside to gamble, saying "We laughed so hard we cried"–a powerful counterpoint to her mother's admonition: "If you laugh too much you'll end up crying."

In the second paradigm, the beloved had expressed the disowned Self *for* the survivor. Unlike the first paradigm in which the beloved made it safe for the survivor to express the forbidden energy herself, in this paradigm the survivor enjoyed the expression of that energy vicariously, by being in a relationship with someone who expressed that energy in her stead. The crisis in bereavement arises from the fact that the death of the beloved leaves the survivor without anyone to express the forbidden, disowned energy for her. The challenge is for the survivor to reclaim and express it for herself.

A major stumbling block in this reclamation process—as is true in all three paradigms—is the fact that expression of the disowned Self is always fraught with danger by definition. It was not for naught that this Self became disowned and tossed into the big black bag in the first place. It is crucial to honor and to process the power of the taboo that led to the disownment, the underlying conflict that led to the banishment of this persona from the whole radiant soul's repertoire.

My work with 40-year-old Betty underscores the importance of processing and honoring the original conflict. Betty's 27-year-old brother Vernon had died of AIDS on our hospice program. Whereas Betty was an obese introvert with multiple serious health problems including a malignancy endangering her very life, Vernon had been "the life of the party." When she was invited to bring to our bereavement group music that expressed the part of Vernon she missed most, Betty chose a tape that included James Brown's "I feel good" and other very upbeat dance music.

After moving to these sounds Betty reported feeling "lighter," "like a ballerina," "so alive." But the original conflict was also re-aroused in all its poignancy. Vernon's life-of-the-party-ness was associated in Betty's mind with the disease that took his life. Betty, as the oldest of a large, single-mother headed family had become the parentified, overresponsible child early in life. Her father, who had not revealed himself to the children as their father until three years before his death twenty years earlier, had left the family for wine and other women—his own version of an exuberant life-of-the-party spirit. For Betty, being the life of the party was, understandably, fraught with danger. Introverted Betty had settled for experiencing her own upbeat, extroverted life force vicariously, through her relationship with Vernon. With Vernon gone and her own health in crisis, Betty's very survival depended on being able to say hello again to her own life-of-the-party persona.

In the third paradigm, the relationship with the beloved had forbidden the survivor to express the disowned Self. It is as though this energy was so hard to control that it required the recruitment of an outside agent to help do the job. Unlike the first two paradigms, in which the relationship with the beloved made some expression of the disownment *possible* for the survivor—either clandestinely or vicariously—in this paradigm the function of the relationship is to insure this energy's repression. The crisis in bereavement in the first two paradigms is that the disownment's *expression* is lost to the survivor. The crisis in this paradigm is that the disownment's *repression* becomes more fragile with the constraining agent buried, so that the "dangerous" energy may become more urgent, more pressing, closer to the surface. The cat's away, the mouse will play—and all hell breaks loose!!

After Rudy died there was no one around to tell Dorothy's Belly Dancer Self, "They're all laughing at you," "Don't make a fool of yourself," or "Not in my back yard." Dorothy was compulsively overeating, gambling, and somewhat suicidal. But the sensuous Bohemian dancer energy persisted, posing an obstinate, formidable and dangerous urge. This 58-year-old housewife from Queens had had an abusive father whose marriage to her mother she blamed on herself, since it was her conception that precipitated their nuptials. Rudy had just been an externalized stand-in for the childhood abuse and self blame that had become so familiar to Dorothy.

We did a life review for Dorothy's Belly Dancer persona. Her origins were in Dorothy's girlhood, in her clandestine trips to Central Park to watch the circus acrobats rehearse, in her love of swimming and gymnastics, and in her clear athletic talent. When asked who wouldn't be surprised to learn that a sensuous Belly Dancer dwelled restlessly in her soul, Dorothy spoke about her maternal grandmother who was also the black sheep in the family, who ran away from Catholic school to live the gypsy life with a circus performer. Dorothy could trace the lineage of this maverick, wild woman spirit!!

Dorothy was of Greek origin, but Rudy's traditional Italian parents lived in the downstairs apartment of their two family home, monitoring her comings and goings and making sure she didn't deviate from the garb and demeanor of the traditional widow's black. A major shift occurred, however, when Dorothy agreed that in addition to the weekly trips to the cemetery where she dutifully "cried hysterically," she would dance a daily dirge for Rudy to express her grief and despair.

Dorothy had had a mastectomy, and now discovered a lump in her second breast. On some level she knew she was dancing for her own life. She danced a belly dance during the last session of our widow's group—fully dressed in costume, makeup, purple veil and bells. She had lost twenty pounds, and had begun going out dancing Friday nights with a girlfriend—sneaking past her in-laws and ignoring her son's disapproval. "I feel like I was let out of jail," she said. And a part of her was! "I want to see if I can have a little happiness before I die." Dorothy had reclaimed, had said hello again, to a lost Self. She had reinhabited a part of her 360° soul.

For the sake of initial clarity, the above three paradigms have been presented as discrete phenomena. In the real world more than one dynamic can and usually do coexist in a single relationship. For example, the beloved who was recruited to help repress the forbidden energy in the other may have simultaneously taken the prerogative of expressing that energy herself. Thus the survivor may be grieving a relationship which both safely kept in check her own expressiveness and gave her the *vicarious* pleasure of that energy's expression.

Often one particular paradigm is the dominant theme in the lost relationship and therefore in the grieving process. However, almost *all* relationships yield rich material when each of the three paradigms are explored. The survivor almost always longs for the treasured way she was seen by the beloved, yearns for the idealized attributes of the deceased, *and* trembles at the possibilities inherent in expressing energies that her relationship with the beloved foreclosed.[11]

The missing of the other, the pain and the loneliness cannot be magically obliterated by this work. But by burying the deceased and only the deceased, by unearthing and resurrecting and reclaiming the survivor's disownments, the survivor can avoid the loneliness and the longing for important parts of Self. The result can be greater wholeness and integration than ever before.

THE PRACTICE

I expect that there will be as many ways of putting these ideas into practice as there are inspired and creative practitioners who may be intrigued by these ideas. My own ways have evolved along with the rest of my professional development. The writings of Michael White and of Hal Stone and Sidra Winkelman[12] contain very satisfying descriptions of their respective methodologies. I have liberally plundered their ideas and mimicked their techniques without shame. There is little value in using this space to try to recapitulate what has already been so ably and definitively expounded elsewhere.

My own synthesis as of this writing includes various tools and techniques that go beyond the traditional perimeters of the talking cure. Individuals differ in the unique way they experience and organize their thoughts, feelings and memories, and in their preferred modes of communication and expression.[13] Since almost all memory has visual, auditory and kinesthetic components,[14] the use of other modalities to augment verbal communication can often afford access to experience that intellect and words alone cannot evoke. The bereavement groups I lead routinely use guided exercises as a springboard (see, e.g., Appendix A) and incorporate music, movement and the visual arts. For example, I may invite bereavement group participants to bring in music that expresses the quality of the beloved they miss most (the second paradigm), to talk about that quality in the group, to drum or sing or move to the music, and then to create a visual image of that quality and of their experience.

By using expressive modalities in addition to traditional verbal ones, greater range of feeling, memory and experience emerge. Another dimension of experience is created, exponentially augmenting the healing effect. The visceral, vibrational experience on a cellular, neurological and muscular level is powerful. The conceptual and verbal modalities are often the place where the self-limiting lies were born, as in "I am not a dancer, my sister is," or "He was the only one who thought I was funny (or sexy or smart)." There may be higher truths in the psyche that are more readily invoked by using experiential modalities and more direct metaphoric communication.[15] By daring to try a new pose, a symbolic gesture or repetitive rhythm, by experimenting with moving or walking the way the beloved did, defenses are sidestepped and possibilities emerge that are beyond the contemplation of the concrete mind and its myths. The soma can have an experience that the knowing brain says died with the beloved. The bereaved can embody a Self that has long ago been tossed into the big bag of disowned, yet treasured energies. A wholeness can be enlivened that our rule-abiding logic said was impossible. Grief for the other can begin when grief for the Self becomes unnecessary.

NOTES

1. Robert Bly, *A Little Book on the Human Shadow.* (San Francisco: Harper-Collins, 1988), 24.

2. Ibid.

3. Hal Stone and Sidra Winkelman, *Embracing Our Selves.* (San Rafael: New World Library, 1989), 3, 27-33.

4. Ibid., 29.

5. Hal Stone and Sidra Winkelman, *Embracing Each Other.* (San Rafael: New World Library, 1989).

6. Stone and Winkelman, *Embracing Our Selves,* 27-33.

7. There are, of course, myriad losses when a loved one dies which are assumed but not enumerated in this article. The focus here is to illuminate an aspect of bereavement that is not often acknowledged.

8. Michael White, "Saying 'Hullo' Again: The Incorporation of the Lost Relationship in the Resolution of Grief," in *Selected Papers.* (Adelaide, South Australia: Dulwich Centre Publications, 1989), 29-30.

9. Peter Marris, *Loss and Change.* (London: Routledge and Kegan Paul, 1986), 32-33.

10. Because the three clients discussed in this article happen to be women, "she" and "her" will be used rather than "he" or "him." The "he or she"/"him

or her" formulation became too cumbersome, but it should be emphasized that these ideas and this work pertain equally to both genders.

11. The negative disownments that inhered in the survivor's relationship with the deceased are an equally fertile area for exploration. The critical eye with which the deceased beheld the survivor, the less than admirable traits of the beloved also yield important information. They bespeak the survivor's self-limiting beliefs. They indicate disowned energies. And they, too, open possibilities for reclamation and greater personal integration.

12. See White, "Saying 'Hullo' Again" and *Narrative Means to Therapeutic Ends* (New York: W.W. Norton & Co., 1990), and Stone and Winkelman, op. cit.

13. Fran J. Levy, ed. *Dance and Other Expressive Art Therapies: When Words Are Not Enough* (New York: Routledge, 1995) xi-xii.

14. Ibid., 42.

15. Ibid., 103.

REFERENCES

Bly, Robert. *A Little Book on the Human Shadow.* San Francisco: HarperCollins, 1988.

Levy, Fran J. ed. *Dance and Other Expressive Art Therapies: When Words are Not Enough.* New York: Routledge, 1995.

Marris, Peter. *Loss and Change.* London: Routledge and Kegan Paul, 1986.

Stone, Hal, and Sidra Winkelman. *Embracing Our Selves.* San Rafael: New World Library, 1989.

_____ . *Embracing Each Other.* San Rafael: New World Library, 1989.

White, Michael. "Saying 'Hullo' Again: The incorporation of the lost relationship in the resolution of grief." Essay in *Selected Papers.* Adelaide, South Australia: Dulwich Centre Publications, 1989.

White, Michael, and David Epston. *Narrative Means to Therapeutic Ends.* New York: W.W. Norton & Company, 1990.

APPENDIX A

Guided Exercise

1. Think about a person you have lost through death, a geographical move, change in the relationship, even a change in the person.

2. What was your relationship with that person? (e.g., parent, spouse, best friend)

   Has this relationship been replaced?

3. What was the explicit function/formal structure of this relationship? (e.g., confidant, shopping buddy, nurturer)

   How do these functions get managed/met in your life now?

4. What quality in this person do you miss most?

   How do you bring that quality into your life now?

   Imagine a gesture, rhythm, way of moving, or a color, piece of music, art or sculpture, a thing in nature that captures or expresses this quality.

5. What quality in you did your lost loved one know/enjoy/appreciate– that others don't recognize or appreciate as fully?

   How do you express that aspect of yourself now?

   Have you let others know about this quality in you?

   When you see yourself through the eyes of this lost loved one, is there a gesture, way of moving, rhythm, color, piece of music, art or sculpture, a thing in nature that captures this cherished way of being seen?

6. In what ways did your relationship with this lost loved one inhibit or constrain you?

   How do you keep a lid on that energy now?

   How do you express that aspect of yourself now?

   Imagine a gesture, pose, way of moving or a color, piece of music, art or sculpture, a thing in nature that captures that quality or energy of yours.

The Interdisciplinary Bereavement Team: Defining and Directing Appropriate Bereavement Care

Barbara L. Bouton

SUMMARY. Hospice bereavement care often occurs in relative isolation from other program components; staff and volunteers are without the guidance, consultation and support provided through the interdisciplinary team that is enjoyed by personnel working in patient care areas. This article promotes a similar interdisciplinary team concept that has been successfully employed in one of the country's largest bereavement programs. Comprised of bereavement program staff, consultants from the patient care program, professional and lay volunteers, this interdisciplinary team defines and directs interventions provided by the bereavement care program. *[Article copies available for a fee from The Haworth Document Delivery Service: 1-800-342-9678. E-mail address: getinfo@haworth.com]*

Barbara L. Bouton, MA, CVA, is Director of Bereavement Care for Hospice of Louisville, where she has worked for over twelve years as a bereavement administrator, volunteer administrator and children's therapist. She is an associate of ACCORD, a national grief education academy, a member of the Interagency Disaster Response Committee in Louisville, Kentucky, a member of NHO's Council of Hospice Professionals and a reviewer with NHO's Educational Material Review Process.

Address correspondence to: Barbara L. Bouton, MA, CVA, Hospice of Louisville, 3532 Ephraim McDowell Drive, Louisville, KY 50205-3224.

[Haworth co-indexing entry note]: "The Interdisciplinary Bereavement Team: Defining and Directing Appropriate Bereavement Care." Bouton, Barbara L. Co-published simultaneously in *The Hospice Journal* (The Haworth Press, Inc.) Vol. 11, No. 4, 1996, pp. 15-24; and: *Bereavement: Client Adaptation and Hospice Services* (ed: Donna Lind Infeld, and Nadine Reimer Penner) The Haworth Press, Inc., 1996, pp. 15-24. Single or multiple copies of this article are available for a fee from The Haworth Document Delivery Service [1-800-342-9678, 9:00 a.m. - 5:00 p.m. (EST). E-mail address: getinfo@ haworth.com].

15

The interdisciplinary team model is essential to hospice care; in fact, it is a required component. To date, it has been an essential component of hospice patient care programs but not of bereavement care programs.

Hospice bereavement care often occurs in relative isolation from other program components. Bereavement staff and volunteers are without the guidance, consultation and support enjoyed by personnel working in patient care areas. Hospice of Louisville has created an interdisciplinary team that provides guidance to professional staff and volunteers providing bereavement care. This interdisciplinary team also helps to define and direct the bereavement care provided by this program, which currently serves over 6,000 family members.

This article will provide a rationale for the establishment of an interdisciplinary hospice bereavement team to provide guidance, consultation and planning for appropriate bereavement intervention. The purpose, composition and process of an effective interdisciplinary bereavement team will be identified. The benefits of utilizing this model, both for the bereavement program and the overall hospice organization, will be highlighted. Finally, considerations for creating an effective interdisciplinary bereavement team for other hospice programs will be identified.

RATIONALE

When the interdisciplinary bereavement team was first proposed for Hospice of Louisville, several questions arose, the answers to which were crucial for ensuring the success of both the proposed team model and the bereavement program. It was important to ask "What do we want to do here?", "What are our goals?" and "What lies within the scope of our bereavement care program and what is clearly beyond the scope of our care?" The discussion of these essential questions helped create definitive boundaries for the scope of bereavement services being provided at that time and more clarity of purpose for the developing interdisciplinary bereavement team.

All hospice programs are confronted with families whose needs fall on a continuum from "very little need" to "extreme need." Hospice programs would do well to define their range of services along that continuum. With such definition, the bereavement program identifies the parameters of its services and responds to the family's needs with more conscientious utilization of resources. How the bereavement program fits into the mission of the organization and contributes to the overall value of the organization are other factors for consideration when setting these parameters. The interdisciplinary bereavement team of Hospice of Louisville was instrumental, particularly during its inception, in determining and setting these parameters.

Given the resources, both personnel and financial, of most hospice bereavement care programs, it is also important for the program to determine what is reasonable and appropriate to provide family members in terms of services and interventions. One of the important determinations Hospice of Louisville's bereavement program made (as a result of the debate, discussion and definition of its interdisciplinary bereavement team) was the differentiation between the provision of bereavement counseling and bereavement therapy. Several authors (Cook and Dworkin, 1992; Worden, 1991) have provided a clear and succinct differentiation that guides the plans and interventions of Hospice of Louisville's bereavement care program. Whereas the goal of grief counseling is to facilitate the tasks of mourning toward successful completion by increasing the reality of the loss, helping the bereaved deal with responses (physical, emotional social and spiritual) to the loss, helping them adapt and adjust and facilitating their reinvestment into life, the goal of bereavement therapy is to identify and resolve the conflicts of separation that prevent completion of these tasks. These distinctions have helped Hospice of Louisville to focus the efforts of its bereavement program upon the provision of counseling and to accept that needs for more intensive intervention are beyond the scope of its program.

This clarity of scope and the parameters within which the bereavement program operates ensure the consistency of bereavement interventions provided. This is true particularly in those programs–like Hospice of Louisville's–where a number of personnel work in the bereavement area. More challenging, perhaps, is determining the specific and practical application of having drawn this line. Naturally, grief issues and other concerns often become juxtaposed with other needs and issues and the ability to separate the two (or more) is questionable. However, an interdisciplinary bereavement team provides a distinct advantage by offering a variety of perspectives from which to make this determination.

The utilization of an interdisciplinary bereavement team also facilitates appropriate referral and follow-up for family members whose needs are beyond the scope of the bereavement program. With the team's involvement and guidance, referral is more likely to happen early on in the family member's grief process and is more likely to be consistent from case to case.

Perhaps the best rationale for the employment of an interdisciplinary bereavement team for Hospice of Louisville's bereavement program has been the opportunities it affords for counseling staff to consult with colleagues about especially complicated and challenging situations. As in the interdisciplinary team model for patient care, the benefit of other perspectives cannot be denied. The presentation of a bereavement case to the team and the ensuing discussion of "What do they want from us?", "What are reasonable and realistic goals for our bereavement program in this situation?" and "What other resources can the family tap into?" provide clear direction for the counselor involved and the bereavement program overall.

Finally, the interdisciplinary bereavement team provides support to the counseling staff providing service as well as to one another. Utilization of an interdisciplinary bereavement team reduces the isolation of bereavement personnel, provides fresh perspectives and support and encourages counseling staff to check out perceptions and counseling strategies.

PURPOSE

Given this rationale for the establishment of an interdisciplinary bereavement team, the purpose of the team can be clearly identified:

1. To ensure the bereavement program is providing interventions that will assist in healthy accommodation to loss
    —by promoting independence, not dependence
    —by attending to how much responsibility staff is taking for meeting the needs of the bereaved versus the amount of responsibility the bereaved is taking.
2. To ensure the bereavement program maintains boundaries it has set for itself, with ongoing evaluation of those
    —by operating within the scope of the program or
    —when operating beyond the scope of the program to recognize the exception, own the exception and address it.
3. To ensure family members receive appropriate and adequate referrals (as indicated).
4. To ensure family members in the program beyond the date of discharge from the hospice program are moving toward closure and/or referral
    —by conscientiously addressing why the bereavement program is still involved, what goals hope to be met, what plans are being made for discharge and whose needs are being met by continued involvement.
5. To provide a forum for philosophical and ethical discussion and debate with respect to the hospice's bereavement program.
6. To provide consultation for bereavement cases assessed to be at high risk for complicated bereavement

—with the goals of facilitating referral and/or identifying clear intervention strategies that fall within the parameters of the bereavement program.

7. To provide consultation for difficult or challenging bereavement cases where family strengths and/or resources may be limited
   —which sometimes means accepting that there is little the bereavement program can to do to meet the family's needs, especially when the needs are extraordinary.
8. To provide consultation for difficult or challenging educational or support group issues.
9. To share ideas, strategies and appropriate therapeutic interventions for bereaved family members.

INTERDISCIPLINARY BEREAVEMENT TEAM COMPOSITION, PROCESS AND MEETINGS

The interdisciplinary bereavement team established at Hospice of Louisville is comprised of bereavement counseling staff (currently three full time counselors); the director of bereavement care; consultants from the patient care program that represent three of hospice's core disciplines (nursing, social work and pastoral care); a bereavement volunteer facilitator (coordinator); several professionals from the community: two therapists in private practice, a therapist from a Jewish family and vocational services agency (who also provides consultation on Jewish tradition, ritual and mourning practices), a funeral home aftercare counselor, a retired chaplain, the coordinator of academic advising for a local community college; and lay bereavement care volunteers (who attend team meetings as their schedules/interests allow).

Essential members for the interdisciplinary bereavement team were identified to be hospice core discipline representatives (nursing, social work, pastoral care and volunteer). Representatives from each of these areas were recruited to the team, with particular efforts directed to those staff persons known to have expertise and interest in bereavement care. The nurse who was recruited has former psychiatric experience, which has been extremely valuable to the team. Assessing the effect of a family member's health on his/her coping, identifying positive and negative effects of medication on a family member's coping as well as the need for a family member to pursue medical treatment have all been issues that have benefitted from this team member's input.

The bereavement care program also felt it would be helpful to recruit persons from outside the hospice whose perspective may be broader and who could lend specific expertise from their areas of practice. Hospice of Louisville was fortunate to have several of these professionals already in its volunteer pool when the team was originated. Since that time new "volunteer professionals" have joined the volunteer program and have either requested serving on the team or recruited for the team.

At the beginning of each team meeting, members in attendance sign a roster that addresses confidentiality issues with the statement: "I understand that all information shared during this team meeting will be kept strictly confidential. I have participated in this meeting for the above named patients/families." Because all team members are either staff or volunteers, they have agreed to abide by the hospice's confidentiality policy.

Currently, Hospice of Louisville's interdisciplinary bereavement team meets bi-weekly in the late afternoon for 1 and 1/2 hour meetings. The time of day for meetings is an important consideration, particularly for staff consultants (who return to the office from the field) and professional volunteers (who leave their workplace to attend meetings).

The interdisciplinary bereavement team's process is similar to a patient care interdisciplinary team, with one notable exception. Because decisions to discuss a case during a team meeting are based on the need for particular focus, attention or consultation, the team enjoys the benefit of taking as much time as is needed to discuss, consider and plan for the care of a particular family or family member. Typically, four to six case presentations are made in each 1 and 1/2 hour meeting.

As would be expected, an initial case presentation (which is made by the bereavement counselor who has assessed the family/family member's bereavement needs) takes the majority of the team's time; update presentations of cases previously discussed generally progress more quickly. To facilitate the team's understanding of the entire family system, bereavement counselors often provide a genogram (McGoldrick and Gerson, 1995) of the family under discussion. In an initial presentation, bereavement counselors use the following format to focus their comments:

Name(s) of the bereaved
Age(s) of the bereaved
Relationship(s) of bereaved to patient
Date of death
Length of patient's illness/length of bereaved's preparation for death
Circumstances of death
Applicable issues/concerns (brief discussion):
    Bereaved's physical health
    Bereaved's emotional expression re: loss
    Bereaved's history of mental health problems

Suspected/confirmed substance abuse in bereaved
Family dynamics (conflict, dysfunction, support, etc.)
Support network of bereaved
Financial concerns
Upheaval/change in living arrangements for bereaved
Nature of relationship between bereaved and deceased
Previous history of loss experiences for bereaved
Suicidal ideation/intent/history of bereaved
Spiritual issues/concerns
Meaningful activities of bereaved (job, hobbies, volunteer work, etc.)

Following the bereavement counselor's presentation, a dynamic and lively discussion ensues (due, in part, to the divergent counseling/therapy orientations of team members) that results in updating the family or family member's plan of care and directing the interventions/strategies to be pursued by the bereavement counselor.

"Update" discussions occur on an "as needed" basis but are scheduled frequently for family members at risk for complication in bereavement or whose coping is of concern. Following a brief account of the team's previous discussion and the plan that was developed, the bereavement counselor brings the team up to date. New issues and concerns are identified. Discussion and the development of a plan to address new problems is completed. In addition to interdisciplinary bereavement team meetings, team members are available to bereavement counselors between meetings when consultation on a particular case is desired or in situations where an outside perspective would be helpful. The team members most often called on for these consultations are, of course, the professional volunteers working in other settings.

BENEFITS OF THE INTERDISCIPLINARY
BEREAVEMENT TEAM

In addition to ensuring the hospice bereavement program provides appropriate and consistent intervention to its clients, the interdisciplinary bereavement team provides several other benefits. Because the team includes representatives of each core hospice discipline (who are also members of other interdisciplinary teams or groups in the patient care program) the bereavement program enjoys increased visibility and credibility that is promoted by these key members throughout the hospice program. The interdisciplinary bereavement team's nurse, social worker and chaplain are more invested in, aware and supportive of bereavement services within their respective departments. The benefit also extends to patients and families served, who are more readily informed about and encouraged to participate in bereavement programs by staff who understand and value bereavement services.

The inclusion of hospice core disciplines and other professionals with various counseling orientations in the bereavement care planning process promotes the same wholistic approach to bereaved families that is a hallmark of hospice patient care. Often, the expertise and unique perspective of a particular discipline or orientation adds a new dimension to the focus of bereavement care for the family.

The existence of the interdisciplinary bereavement team also ensures accountability of the bereavement program and its personnel, who are expected to address issues and pursue counseling goals as identified and directed by the team. In the few instances where, with a change in circumstances or additional information, a plan of care needs to be altered, the bereavement counselor returns to the team for further discussion and planning. This also ensures that the counseling goals being pursued are realistic, sound and consistent from family to family.

The support provided to personnel of the bereavement program is one of the benefits most valued by bereavement counselors at Hospice of Louisville. A high level of trust has developed within the team and, as a result, staff are comfortable discussing their strengths, weaknesses and vulnerabilities. Counselors openly ask their questions and seek input that will not only enable them to provide quality care for bereaved family members but also to increase their skills and expertise. The cohesive, genuine "team" spirit and willingness of the group to take responsibility for the care they direct increases the confidence of bereavement program staff and of the program overall. Having considered the input of all team members, there is increased confidence that the program has considered all perspectives and decisions regarding bereavement intervention are "owned" by the team. The group process that leads to those decisions is respected and valued.

Finally, the work of the interdisciplinary bereavement team benefits lay volunteers, who are encouraged to attend team meetings. Attendance provides great learning opportunities, especially for the unseasoned volunteer who has an opportunity to increase his/her bereavement skills repertoire. Participation in the interdisciplinary bereavement team also provides clarity about the roles of bereavement counseling and volunteer staff, the goals of the bereavement care program and their own supportive interventions. Additionally, the camaraderie and support of the team enhances the volunteers' experience and facilitates their sense of belonging and contributing.

REPLICATION OF THIS MODEL

Perhaps the most challenging aspect of creating an interdisciplinary bereavement team such as the one described here is the recruitment of counseling/therapy professionals on a volunteer basis. Hospice of Louisville has found the inclusion of these team members to be vital to the success of the interdisciplinary bereavement team, as their perspective is such an objective, yet wholistically therapeutic, one. These professionals, in contrast to what might be expected, are highly motivated to participate in such a forum and have found that the team model meets some of their needs as well. As several of the professionals on Hospice of Louisville's interdisciplinary bereavement team work in private practice or other isolated situations, they, too, are denied the benefits of collaboration, connection and support from colleagues. The interdisciplinary bereavement team has clearly helped to fill this need for these practitioners. The team makes an ongoing practice of distributing helpful resource articles, information about conferences or continuing educational programs available, thus adding more value to the team experience for all members. As an example, the chaplain consultant has also developed and coordinates a "musicare" program for hospice patients/families. On a monthly basis, she brings musical resources with a death, dying or bereavement theme to the team meeting. This practice not only enhances the learning and experience of all team members, but promotes the "musicare" program and increases team members' awareness of innovative approaches to patient and bereavement care.

Statistics indicate that people are willing to volunteer when they are asked; and when clear, manageable opportunities that make a positive and visible difference are presented, people respond. One of the professional volunteers who serves on the team even received the approval and support of her organization's management to participate on Hospice of Louisville's interdisciplinary bereavement team, as the opportunity was viewed as a community outreach effort of the agency. Now that the interdisciplinary bereavement team of Hospice of Louisville is well established and enjoys a good reputation, staff and other professional volunteers have requested joining/serving on the team.

In short, the creation of an interdisciplinary bereavement team to define and direct the care of a hospice bereavement program is relatively simple. Identification of key member roles is a critical first step. Initial meetings are well spent in discussion of the rationale for creating the team, determining its purposes and identifying the practical processes it will follow. Concurrently, of course, it will serve the bereavement program well to define its scope and the parameters of services it will provide. Doing so provides all team members with a foundation upon which recommendations that are clear, consistent and within the goals of the program can be made.

It has been the intent of this article to promote the concept of an interdisciplinary bereavement team to define and direct the provision of bereavement services for a hospice program. Utilization of a team model such as this assures that the bereavement services provided to family members are clear, consistent, responsible and facilitate their healthy accommodation to loss.

REFERENCES

Cook, Alicia Skinner and Dworkin, Daniel S. (1992). *Helping the Bereaved: Therapeutic Interventions for Children, Adolescents and Adults.* USA, Basic Books.
McGoldrick, Monica and Gerson, Randy (1985). *Genograms in Family Assessment.* New York, W.W. Norton and Company, Inc.
National Hospice Organization (1993). *Standards of a Hospice Program of Care.* Arlington, Virginia, National Hospice Organization.
Worden, J. William (1991). Grief Counseling and Grief Therapy—*A Handbook for the Mental Health Practitioner*; Second Edition. New York, Springer Publishing Company.

Bereavement Services Development in a Rural Setting

Herbert I. Wilker
Ben Lowell

SUMMARY. Functioning as a hospital-based hospice program of a large medical center, bereavement services are not limited to hospice families in one location. Bereavement services are offered to those who died within the medical center and to the residents of the three county area the hospice serves. This paper identifies ways to offer bereavement follow-up to hospice and non-hospice families. This will include discussion of mixing together survivors of different types of death in a support group atmosphere. Due to the smaller population of a rural setting, the need to be creative to offer bereavement services to the community is imperative. This paper will discuss how our Bereavement Services have expanded in response to the needs of the communities in the three county area we serve. We will discuss survey results, meeting and support group data used to generate supporting information to allow our services to grow.

Learning objectives for this article consist of readers being able to identify ways to develop and expand bereavement services; incorporating various types of death in a support group setting; and ways to better serve non-hospice families in need of bereavement follow-up. Topics include a description of Bereavement Services; Pre-Death

Herbert I. Wilker, MSW, LSW, is a Bereavement Counselor at St. Rita's Hospice. Ben Lowell, MDiv, is Hospice Chaplain with St. Rita's Hospice.

Address correspondence to: Herbert I. Wilker, MSW, LSW, St. Rita's Hospice, 730 West Market Street, Lima OH 45801.

[Haworth co-indexing entry note]: "Bereavement Services Development in a Rural Setting." Wilker, Herbert I. and Ben Lowell. Co-published simultaneously in *The Hospice Journal* (The Haworth Press, Inc.) Vol. 11, No. 4, 1996, pp. 25-39; and: *Bereavement: Client Adaptation and Hospice Services* (ed: Donna Lind Infeld, and Nadine Reimer Penner) The Haworth Press, Inc., 1996, pp. 25-39. Single or multiple copies of this article are available for a fee from The Haworth Document Delivery Service [1-800-342-9678, 9:00 a.m. - 5:00 p.m. (EST). E-mail address: getinfo@haworth.com].

Bereavement Intervention; Open and Closed Support groups; Routine Bereavement Follow-up of Hospice families; Quarterly Nursing Home Staff Support groups; Widow/Widower Brunch Social; opportunities to educate the community about Death/Dying; and data collection for Bereavement Needs. *[Article copies available for a fee from The Haworth Document Delivery Service: 1-800-342-9678. E-mail address: getinfo@haworth.com]*

St. Rita's Medical Center Hospice functions as a hospital-based hospice program. Bereavement services are offered to survivors of loved ones who died within the Medical Center and to the residents of the surrounding, rural three-county hospice service area. We will present material enabling readers to identify creative ways to offer bereavement follow-up to hospice and non-hospice families. This will include discussion of combining survivors of different types of death in support group settings. Due to the smaller population of a rural setting, the need to be creative in offering bereavement services is imperative. We will describe how our bereavement services have expanded to meet the needs of the communities in the three-county area and present survey results and support group information which generated data to justify growth of our services.

DEMOGRAPHIC INFORMATION

St. Rita's Medical Center is a 424-bed, regional medical center serving a 10-county, mostly rural, region with a population of over 466,000. The medical center is located near downtown Lima, Ohio. Lima has a population of 47,827 and is located 70 miles from Toledo, Columbus and Dayton, OH and Ft. Wayne, IN.

St. Rita's Hospice program began in 1983. The daily patient census grew from less than ten during the 1980s, to approximately 45 patients in 1995. St. Rita's Hospice primarily serves the residents of three counties: Allen, Auglaize and Putnam counties in west central Ohio, and fourteen nursing homes within these three counties and Mercer County. The cultural makeup of the residents in these counties are primarily white and German heritage descent.

HISTORICAL FOCUS

The bereavement services of St. Rita's were initially coordinated by a Licensed Practical Nurse (LPN) who also worked as the Volunteer Coordinator. Post-death follow-up was primarily done with mailings, involving very little personal contact. A social worker was available through the Medical Center's Social Services department, on a referral basis, for social work concerns.

Based on a recommendation from the Joint Commission on Accreditation of Healthcare Organizations survey team in 1990, a full-time social worker was hired to do hospice social work. A bereavement team was created to address the needs and high risk factors of grievers. The team consisted of a volunteer/bereavement coordinator, a hospice chaplain and a social worker. The master's prepared social worker assumed responsibility for most of the complicated bereaved clients. During this time, the hospice nurses completed bereavement assessments. St. Rita's Hospice also instituted a memorial service to supplement the Medical Center's memorial services.

During 1992, the responsibilities of the bereavement services coordinator were included in the job description of the hospice social worker. Subsequently, the bereavement team was made up of the social worker and the chaplain. Nurses were no longer required to complete bereavement assessments, as the bereavement team assumed these duties. Bereavement follow-up contacts became more regular and frequent. In August 1993, the first monthly bereavement support group, "Free To Grieve," was held. It was offered to the surrounding communities and to the local prison population.

St. Rita's Hospice initiated use of a bereavement packet developed as a result of a joint venture between St. Rita's Medical Center and another local hospital, Lima Memorial. Quality assurance was conducted by documentation and chart review. Patient satisfaction surveys were also completed on Hospice services.

As a result of changes in the social worker staff member, the Hospice chaplain played a vital and pivotal part in the development of the bereavement services. The chaplain experienced many changes in the staffing and delivery of bereavement follow-up. The stable and consistent role he provided allowed for a period of growth, development and a connection to the past.

SURVEY OF BEREAVEMENT NEEDS

During 1994, long-term goals for expanding bereavement services were established and data was generated to assess bereavement needs in the targeted communities. In April 1994, a formal proposal was submitted to the Vice President of Mission Services for St. Rita's Medical Center, describing the need for expansion of bereavement services offered by St. Rita's Hospice. Data to justify expansion came from several sources. Initially, a written inquiry about bereavement concerns was mailed to local funeral directors, but this yielded little response. Next, telephone contacts were made to facilitators of established grief-related groups in the communities to explore what services were already being provided. We learned that various churches and funeral homes offered monthly or biweekly support groups for adults only. Two organized formal groups for children were offered but were located seventy miles apart. Subsequent planning meetings were held and during November 1994, St. Rita's Hospice sent a survey to pastors, doctors and mental health agencies to assess bereavement needs in the community. Five hundred and forty surveys were mailed. Fifteen surveys were undeliverable.

Of 375 surveys mailed to pastors, 75 were completed for a 20 percent return rate. Of 127 surveys mailed to doctors, 42 were completed for a 33 percent return rate. Targeted specialties included: internal medicine, family practice, oncology, surgery, psychology, psychiatry, urology, cardiology, neurology, pulmonology, infection specialists, pediatrics, and others who referred patients to Hospice in the past.

Of 23 surveys mailed to mental health agencies, five were completed for a 22 percent return rate. One survey was sent to each agency in the area. Five questions were on the survey:

1. What percentage of clients each week seek help for grief-related symptoms?
2. What percentage of clients each week seek assistance in their adjustment to deaths?
3 a. Do you offer formal bereavement services?
    b. If so, check all that apply.
4. Are bereavement needs being met?
5. Would you use a bereavement referral source if one was available?

Figures 1-5 show the responses to each question by group.

SURVEY RESULTS

The responses to our survey indicated that a small percentage (less than 25%) of respondent's clients seek help due to grief-related symptoms or identify having difficulty adjusting to a death. This was common among

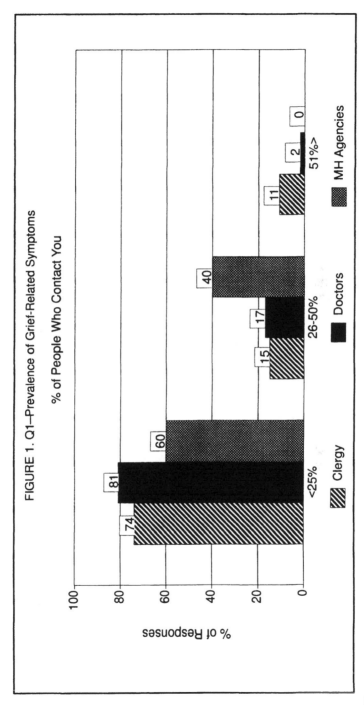

FIGURE 1. Q1--Prevalence of Grief-Related Symptoms

29

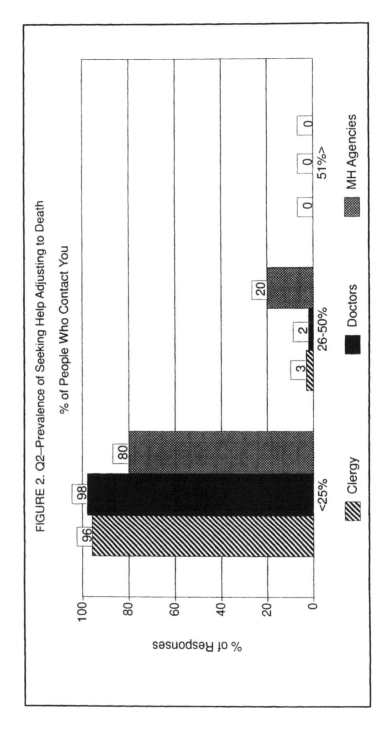

FIGURE 2. Q2–Prevalence of Seeking Help Adjusting to Death

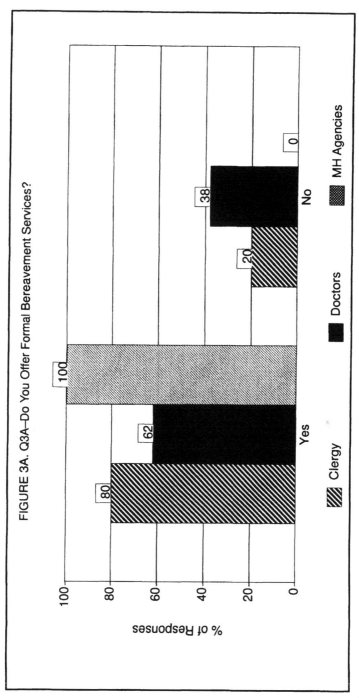

FIGURE 3A. Q3A—Do You Offer Formal Bereavement Services?

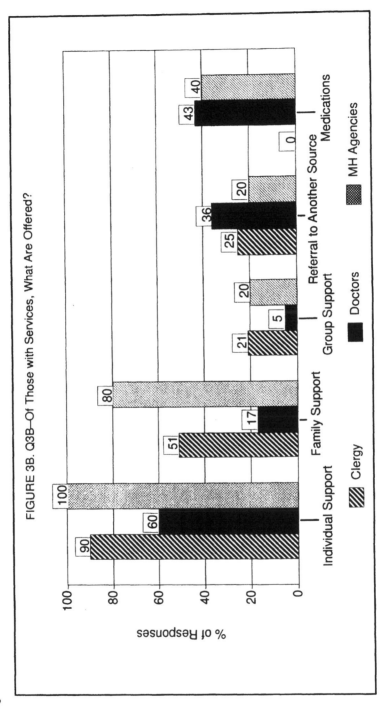

FIGURE 3B. Q3B—Of Those with Services, What Are Offered?

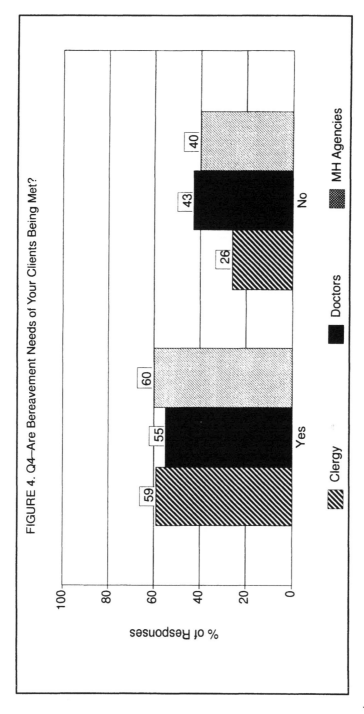

FIGURE 4. Q4–Are Bereavement Needs of Your Clients Being Met?

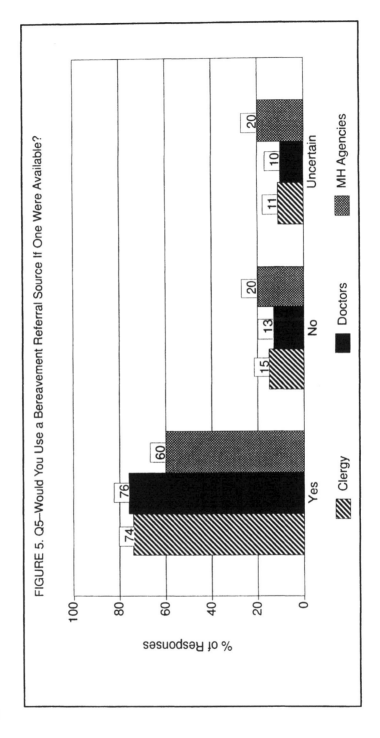

FIGURE 5. Q5—Would You Use a Bereavement Referral Source If One Were Available?

the three targeted groups surveyed. We anticipated finding higher percentages of clients with these experiences.

The survey results indicate that all three targeted groups offer some type of formal bereavement services, with clergy and Mental Health agencies ranking higher (80% and 100% respectively) than doctors (62%). Twenty percent of clergy and 38% of doctors indicated they do not offer formal bereavement services. One response from a Mental Health agency added "We address grief issues in our services, but only in a broad sense. We do not specialize or focus on grief, therefore, I think a specialized service would be excellent."

Of those survey respondents offering formal bereavement services, specific services were identified. The most common service offered by all three groups was individual support. Family support was the next most frequently offered service by clergy and Mental Health agencies, while medication was the second highest formal bereavement service offered by doctors. Group support was offered at a lower rate in all three groups, however, referrals to another source were made more often. Referral sources identified were: local hospices, local counselors or psychologists, YWCA support groups, or peer loss groups. Surprisingly, a large number of doctors and Mental Health agencies offered medications to clients (43% and 40% respectively).

Assessing whether the bereavement needs of clients are being met adequately, over half of all three groups responded "yes," while 26% of clergy, 43% and 40% of doctors and Mental Health agencies respectively reported "no." Some participants shared they were "not sure" or "for the most part depends on the situation," and "there is always room for improvement." One pastor shared that "In this traditional German-American village, people don't readily admit or discuss their problems–a lot of 'yep' and 'nope', but little elaboration is the rule." Although over half of the responses showed that bereavement needs are being met, there is uncertainty whether enough support is offered to allow for grief work.

The last area of our survey focused on the potential demand for a bereavement referral source. The response was clearly favorable, as 74% of clergy, 76% of doctors and 60% of Mental Health agencies reportedly would use one. Of those who responded "no" or "uncertain," many of their written responses were concerned about the qualifications of the person offering the bereavement support or "if it is consistent with biblical principles." Others were uncertain, expressing interest depending on the situation or referring to the availability of adequate bereavement resources. Many shared that such a source would enhance the services already available in the communities.

From the results of this survey and the frequent incoming telephone calls inquiring of bereavement services/groups and educational inservices, we at St. Rita's Hospice have expanded our services to begin addressing many of the identified bereavement needs.

EXPANSION OF SERVICES

Before the fall of 1994, St. Rita's Hospice sponsored and facilitated an ongoing, monthly bereavement adult support group called, "Free to Grieve." This group was successful, based on the average number of participants and the amount of support offered. In the fall of 1994, our first five-week closed group series for adults, "Grief Journeys," was offered in Lima. We publicized by mail, flyers, and the media (local television and newspaper). We chose to meet for five weeks for various reasons. A five-week series allows us to offer the support group in other communities quicker and we were concerned that residents may not commit themselves to a longer series. Group bonding and support between members were established during the earlier meetings and many chose to sign-up for a telephone list to call others after the series ended.

The participants' evaluations of the group are favorable. During the last meeting of "Grief Journeys," each participant received an evaluation to rate the quality of the support group. On a numeric scale (5 representing excellent and 1 representing poor), most of the participants' evaluation responses are near the excellent rating. The participants evaluate the educational presentation; packets of reading information; format of group and of series; room environment; time and day of meeting and small group discussions. All participants are encouraged to give written feedback, especially identifying areas for improvement.

Group enrollment is not restricted based on the type of death (natural, accidental, suicidal or homicidal) (Worden) the survivors experience. Due to the smaller number of participants in rural settings, restricting group membership would greatly reduce the size of our groups. After running these groups for one year, we observed people are able to extend emotional support to one another. Bringing the survivors of different types of death together does not greatly deter the bonding between members. During the first meeting we identify the different types of deaths and educate the participants on the different reactions they may experience [(Rando) (Worden)]. An overview of the group, introduction of staff, discussion of goals, and weekly agenda are also addressed during the first meeting. During subsequent groups, additional education on grief, mourning and various exercises (relaxation techniques, coping skills) are offered to assist the participants' adjustment to the deaths. Occasionally, we will have a previous group participant share from his/her grief experiences and the group process.

During the summer of 1995, we offered our first five-week children's group series, "WINGs" (Within Normal Grief). We publicized the group through mailings, flyers and the local television station. The number of families to register was small (four) and only two families committed to attend the group. Interest in the group was favorable yet the timing of the group was poor due to the busy summer schedules of many families. During the announcement of "WINGs," many inquiries regarding a "Younger Widows/Widowers" group were received. Numerous younger widowed adults had a strong need to be with others of similar age, but were reluctant to attend "Grief Journeys."

In September 1995, the first younger widowed group was held in Lima. The ongoing, two-hour group meets on the second and fourth Thursday of each month and is open to anyone 45 years old or younger who experienced the death of a spouse (Nudel). The group offers grief education and time for sharing. The group is very fortunate to have the participation and the experience of a woman whose husband died seven years ago. She serves as a "role model" in the group, offering insights and guidance to the "newly" widowed. The group process provides opportunities for her to rework some grief issues, also.

During 1995, we offered a weekly, informal brunch group at a local restaurant for support to widows/widowers. This group was intended to reach adults who were not working and were unable to attend one of our evening groups. The membership of the group with a core of six individuals remained intact through the year. The majority of attendees are women. One of the consistent factors in all of our support groups is the small number of men who attend. It continues to be a challenge to find ways to encourage men to attend support groups, even with men facilitators.

Another ongoing grief support group St. Rita's Hospice now offers is to the staff of some contracting nursing homes. These quarterly meetings are held at the facilities. The groups allow nursing home staff opportunities to learn about grief and to share experiences related to their residents' deaths and personal deaths.

Through use of quality assurance (by chart reviews and patient satisfaction surveys), St. Rita's Hospice initiated a more formalized process to assess anticipatory grief and death education needs. While death issues are addressed during the initial psychosocial assessment, we believe it is important to have an established form to allow for consistency in exploring these issues. The Anticipatory Grief and Death Education Assessment (see

Appendix I) collects important information for the identification of high-risk bereavement factors and allows us to tailor our bereavement follow-up program to address bereavement concerns quicker.

Since the fall of 1994, St. Rita's Bereavement Services have expanded to better meet the grief needs of the communities served. Survey responses from pastors, doctors, mental health agencies and inquiries from communities about the availability of grief support groups led us in the current direction. We feel the multi-dimensional program has significantly improved St. Rita's ability to meet a broad array of bereavement needs.

AUTHOR NOTE

Herbert I. Wilker, MSW, LSW, received his Master of Social Work from the Ohio State University, Columbus, Ohio in June 1993. Mr. Wilker has eight years of Hospice Social Work experience and Bereavement Counseling from the Hospice of Dayton, and St. Rita's Medical Center's Hospice Program, in Lima, Ohio. Mr. Wilker has experiences in coordinating and facilitating various bereavement groups, offering grief education and counseling to individuals and families. Since his employment with St. Rita's Medical Center's Hospice Program, Bereavement Services have expanded to the residents of the three county area served by Hospice. Also, Mr. Wilker has taught a Death/Dying course at Edison Community College in Piqua, Ohio.

Ben Lowell, MDiv., has been a United Methodist minister for seventeen years. His work with Hospice began in 1989, at St. Rita's Medical Center Hospice Program in Lima, Ohio. As a chaplain, he finds himself working with patients and families during the patient's illness. His role continues with our families in the area of bereavement. He keeps in touch with our families by phone, visits, memorial services and with support groups. This is a very rewarding area of ministry and is a natural follow-up, in many instances, from meeting them while the patient was alive. Ben also does a number of funerals for our patients.

Portions of this paper were presented at the National Hospice Organization's National Conference Series on Spiritual/Bereavement/Psychosocial Aspects of Hospice Care–San Francisco, CA, August, 1995.

BIBLIOGRAPHY

Nudel, Adele. (1986). *Starting Over: Help for Young Widows and Widowers.* New York: Dodd, Mead Co.

Rando, T.A. (1993). *Treatment of Complicated Mourning.* Champaign, IL: Research Press.

Worden, J. William (1991). *Grief Counseling and Grief Therapy.* New York: Springer Publishing Company.

APPENDIX I. St. Rita's Hospice Program
Anticipatory Grief and Death Education Assessment

I. Explore with the patient/caregiver significant deaths in their lives:

_____

_____

A. What impact did these deaths have in their lives?

_____

_____

B. What issues remain unresolved (unfinished business)?

_____

_____

II. What meaning or purpose does death have in patient/caregivers lives? How is death viewed?

_____

_____

A. What source of regrets/guilt feelings are identified?

_____

_____

B. Has there been pre-planning or discussion of the death of patient/caregiver? (DPOA, Will, Living Will, Funeral Arrangements)

_____

_____

C. What risk factors are identified for potential complicated adjustment?

_____

_____

Meeting the Bereavement Needs
of Kids in Patient/Families–
Not Just Playing Around

Kathleen Muleady Seager
Susan C. Spencer

SUMMARY. Children grieve differently than adults. Although the unit of care in hospice is the patient and family, emphasis is often on the grown members of the family and the anticipatory grief and bereavement needs of children and adolescents are sometimes not met adequately. In this paper, hands-on strategies for working with children both before and after a significant death are presented, as well as appropriate context information on the grieving process for youth under age 18. *[Article copies available for a fee from The Haworth Document Delivery Service: 1-800-342-9678. E-mail address: getinfo@haworth. com]*

Kathleen Muleady Seager, MA, is currently affiliated with Teleios Counseling Services, Cedar Falls, IA. Kate has been affiliated with Cedar Valley Hospice and previously held the positions of Counselor and Coordinator of Grief Support Services there. Kate holds a masters degree in counseling and is a Fellow and Diplomate of the American Board of Medical Psychotherapists. Susan C. Spencer, BSW, MEd, is Youth Services Specialist with Cedar Valley Hospice, Waterloo, IA. Susan coordinates the Youth Support Services and Katie and Quincy Koala Programs and provides resources and consultation to staff and the community regarding the grief related needs of youth under 18. Susan also provides counseling and play therapy to children dealing with serious or terminal illness or in grief.

Address correspondence to: Kathleen Muleady Seager, Teleios Counseling Services, 3914 Heritage Road, Cedar Falls, IA 50613.

[Haworth co-indexing entry note]: "Meeting the Bereavement Needs of Kids in Patient/Families–Not Just Playing Around." Seager, Kathleen Muleady, and Susan C. Spencer. Co-published simultaneously in *The Hospice Journal* (The Haworth Press, Inc.) Vol. 11, No. 4, 1996, pp. 41-66; and: *Bereavement: Client Adaptation and Hospice Services* (ed: Donna Lind Infeld, and Nadine Reimer Penner) The Haworth Press, Inc., 1996, pp. 41-66. Single or multiple copies of this article are available for a fee from The Haworth Document Delivery Service [1-800-342-9678, 9:00 a.m. - 5:00 p.m. (EST). E-mail address: getinfo@haworth.com].

INTRODUCTION

The unit of care in hospice is the patient and the family, with family being defined creatively at times according to the relationships of the patient to his/her biological family and circle of support. Within this circle of significant persons, for most patients, will be children or adolescents.

While the typical hospice patient is of Medicare age, life threatening conditions or disease process can affect anyone. Therefore, every hospice will have children and young adults, as well as seniors, as patients at some time. Children who are living with patients, whether as siblings, children or grandchildren, or who have close ties to patients, will be profoundly affected by the impending death, and they will grieve. It is essential that the individual anticipatory grief and bereavement needs of these young people be met in the care provided to the family by the hospice interdisciplinary team.

Children grieve differently than adults. Their understanding of the world and their ability to comprehend death changes as they grow and move through different developmental stages. Clear and accurate communication appropriate to their level of comprehension and unconditional listening and affection are critical in shepherding children through this potentially traumatic time. As children are largely unable to articulate their fears, feelings and needs, it becomes our responsibility as adults to provide them with the venues to express themselves and work through issues which could later become problems if not adequately addressed at the time.

One does not need to be a trained play therapist to communicate with and provide this support to children. Most youth in patient/families are able to deal with death and move through their grief in a healthy manner as long as they are given the support and opportunity to do so. One of the first steps is to educate the family as to what to expect and what is normal in children's reactions to impending death and grief. Children will model their responses largely on the adults around them. If the grown-ups are falling apart, they'll get the message, "This is bad, we are falling apart!", but if the adults project a message that "This really hurts and we are sad but we will be OK," the children will follow suit.

Presented below is the essential background information for understanding the bereavement needs of youth, followed by intervention strategies any qualified hospice human services professional should be able to utilize. Also included is a bibliography of books and other materials to be used with children and adolescents.

AGES AND STAGES

Interest from hospices and human service agencies in dealing with children's bereavement concerns has been increasing throughout the country. As more literature has been produced defining the concepts children possess about death at different developmental levels and the behaviors that they often exhibit at these levels, more strategies and techniques have been developed to help these children cope with death and grief.

The "ages and stages" concept of death understanding has been criticized by Corr (1995) as not taking into account that every child is singular and unique in his/her perceptions, reactions, cognitive abilities, emotional maturity, etc. Few people would disagree with this. However, those working with children need some commonality standards and norms to use in reassuring parents and significant adults that their child is behaving or grieving normally. Even more importantly, norms are needed for use in assessments and in making recommendations for more intense counseling, when appropriate.

A child's ability to understand the concept of death and what it means to him/her varies with the child's age. Adults need to be aware of the level of understanding of the child and adjust any explanation to that level. The most important thing to remember is to be as accurate, honest, and open as possible. Do not give elaborate explanations. Giving more information than he/she can understand only confuses the child. Encourage questions and assure the child that any emotions he/she feels are the same feelings other children have had in similar situations.

Children and adolescents do not grieve in a linear pattern as adults are more likely to do. How far they are able to progress in understanding and accepting a death and moving through the grief process is limited by their developmental stage (Corr 1995; Grollman 1990; Papenbrock & Voss 1988; Schaefer & Lyons 1993). Therefore, children often grieve in a clumping pattern of sometimes intense periods separated by long intervals where they apparently are not affected by the loss. This pattern is often misunderstood by parents/significant adults and schools who are unlikely to associate an appearance of acting out behavior and diminished attention in a fourth grader to the death of his father two years earlier. Some examples may help to demonstrate this phenomenon.

Alyssa was three and one half years of age when her father died in a car accident. When she initially balked at beginning kindergarten two years later, her mother assumed it was normal apprehension at something new. However, when the child was unable to adjust and also began suddenly speaking of the death of her father and having nightmares, the family requested she be assessed by the hospice grief staff. In the play room,

Alyssa demonstrated she had several issues to work through concerning the loss of her father. These were things she was not developmentally able to address earlier.

Kyle was the middle of three boys when his father died of cancer on a hospice program. His two year old brother regressed from walking to crawling, his seven year old older sibling started trying to fill his father's role as "head of the household" and Kyle, at five, seemed totally unaffected by the death. The next year, however, as the family had moved through their grief in a generally open and healthy manner, Kyle suddenly became, as his mother put it, out of control. It was now his time and turn to grieve.

After Terrie's father died of a brain tumor under hospice care when she was thirteen, she received some intense counseling from the grief staff. As the youngest child and only girl, she had had a special relationship as "Daddy's little girl." Terrie progressed well and appeared to be functioning healthily and normally after the year anniversary of the death. Then, one evening when she was sixteen, the hospice on-call nurse received a frantic call from Terrie's mother. Terrie had tried on her prom dress, burst into tears and locked herself in the bathroom, crying hysterically and screaming for her father. Intervention by a grief counselor revealed Terrie had suddenly been hit with the realization that Dad was not there to see her "all grown up." Some short term counseling assisted Terrie through this crisis and she and her mother were prepared for the likelihood that other developmental milestones such as graduation, marriage, even the birth of her children, would also be likely to produce a grief upsurge, and this was normal.

The following developmental outline should be used as a guideline and not interpreted as hard and fast rules. Emotionally and cognitively, all of the following age groups may exhibit irritability, anxiety, lowered self esteem, apathy, depression, feelings of rejection, distractibility, short attention spans, and a decline in school work or usual ability to attend to a task or play.

A CHILD'S UNDERSTANDING OF DEATH (based on Corr 1995; Grollman 1990; Papenbrock & Voss 1988; Schaefer & Lyons 1993)

Under two years of age:

- Can sense that something is different, that there is a change in the emotional atmosphere
- Does not understand yet what death is
- Probably won't remember the person who died

- Needs a lot of nonverbal communication (i.e., hugs, rocking, continued routine)
- Acting out behaviors include:
  fussiness, clinginess to adults, regression

Three to five years of age:

- Sees death as temporary, believes that the person will return or can be visited
- Has difficulty handling concepts such as heaven, the soul or spirit
- Feels sadness, but often for only a short time and often escapes into play, giving adults the impression the child isn't really grieving
- Substitutes attachment to another person in exchange for attachment to person who died
- May not remember the person who died
- Needs a daily routine, structure, affection, and reassurance
- Acting out behaviors include:
  regression, nightmares, aggression, non-compliance

Five to nine years of age:

- Begins to understand that death is final and permanent
- Begins to have a fear of death and of others dying
- May feel guilt (magical thinking) and blame self for the death
- Has difficulty putting problems and feelings into words
- Often asks concrete and specific questions about the death, the body, etc.
- Identifies strongly with the deceased
- Acting out behaviors include:
  compulsive caregiving, aggression, possessiveness, regression, headaches, stomachaches, phobias

Ten to twelve years of age:

- Recognizes that death is inevitable and irreversible
- May view death as a punishment
- Retains some elements of magical thinking
- Often very curious and interested in the "gory" details
- May come up with own theories or explanations of the reasons for the death
- May have many practical questions about the body, the funeral, etc.

- Acting out behaviors include:
  aggression, possessiveness, headaches, stomachaches, phobias, defiance

Thirteen to eighteen years of age:

- Nearing adult levels of concepts
- May worry or think about own death
- Often avoids discussions of death
- Fears "looking different"
- May question religious beliefs
- Often angry at the deceased
- May fear the future
- Acting out behaviors include:
  aggression, possessiveness, headaches, stomachaches, phobias, increased sexual activity, increased drug use, increased risk-taking, defiance, suicidal ideation.

COMMUNICATING WITH CHILDREN

Quite often human service professionals are taught to communicate effectively with adults, but few are taught any specific techniques to enhance communication with children. We have determined four goals in communicating with children (Spencer, NHO Conference, 1995): (1) to establish rapport, (2) to determine the child's developmental level, (3) to speak to the child at that level, and (4) to form evaluations based on the child's responses. Once these goals are accomplished, the adult can begin to determine the child's needs and help that child develop coping strategies.

Establishing rapport is a little more complicated than just being able to "get down on the floor with a child" (Grollman, NHO conference, 1995), although this is a wonderful start. A child needs to be met where they are at the time. If a child is digging worms in the garden, then the adult should be digging worms in the garden. If a child is building with blocks, then the adult needs to be taking an interest in the blocks. Children do not want to be taken away from an already established activity to join a total stranger in a different room on adult-sized furniture. A nonthreatening location (a playroom, the child's own room, a relative's home) is a good place to start.

Trying to establish rapport through eye contact may not necessarily work with a child. Most of us are taught to maintain eye contact with adults to encourage the other to speak and to let the other know we are interested in what they are saying. Children can view eye contact as a threat, as the times children get the most eye contact are when they are in trouble. Often a parent is nose to nose with them saying, "If you don't stop teasing your brother, you're grounded for a month," or a teacher stares at a child while saying, "Jenny, would you like to share that note with the whole class?" Joining a child in an activity is much more effective than eye contact. Some of the best counseling sessions can occur while playing with play dough, drawing, or kicking a soccer ball around a field.

Another step in establishing rapport with a child is to be comfortable with silence. Counselors are trained to allow silence with an adult to allow the client to formulate a thought or work up the courage to share something important and possibly revealing. Children can be silent for many reasons. Some can be shy and are not ready to talk. Some may not be ready to reveal a thought or emotion, or the child may not have the vocabulary to express himself or herself.

Many children fall into silences during play/counseling sessions and the counselor may not know exactly why. To the child, the room may not be silent at all as he/she fills it with imaginary sounds or people. When the child is ready to break away from the invented world, he/she will quite often bring a statement back from that illusory neverland that is revealing and furthers the counseling process.

Rapport can never be established if the counselor does not consistently attempt to be open and honest with a child. Children recognize fakes. They identify insincerity and evasiveness, and they quite often point them out to the adult. Honesty from a grown-up encourages children to relax and reveal their feelings and problems. As with an adult, body gestures and facial expressions from the counselor which indicate interest and acceptance can encourage a child to relax and open up to the processing of difficult emotions.

Determining the child's level of understanding is easily accomplished by talking with them, usually about safe subjects such as their family, school, pets, etc. A nine-year-old who talks "baby talk" will need explanations geared to his obviously younger level of communication ability. An exceptionally bright and precocious 5-year old might be able to understand words or explanations beyond the range of her fellow kindergartners. There are no set rules in ascertaining a child's level of understanding. Adults need to rely on their instincts in making as accurate a determination as possible.

Once the level of understanding has been determined, the adult begins speaking to the child at that level. Most counselors know immediately if they have assessed the child's level correctly. A child who begins to look as if the counselor is speaking Greek has not been accurately evaluated. Even more common than looking confused is the child who totally turns off and begins to look around the room, out the window, or at the floor. The child may even look bored and yawn–a sure sign the adult has passed the child's level of understanding. Expectations and vocabulary need to be lowered.

Once the adult is successfully speaking at a child's level of understanding and an interchange is going on, the counselor tries to make an assessment of the child based on the child's statements, body language, and play. At best, such evaluations are educated guesses sprinkled with a heavy dose of common sense. Often the adult deduces correctly and the child progresses further in coping with the problem. Many a good counselor has made a guess about a child's feelings, attitudes or emotional state, only to have the child indignantly and honestly correct them. Either way, progress is being made toward identifying the underlying problems and helping the child develop coping strategies.

CONCEPTS OF PLAY THERAPY

Many of the techniques presented here are based on play therapy strategies. This paper does not suffice to teach play therapy, as one article is not a substitute for formal training and supervised clinical hours. However, the basic techniques and concepts of play therapy are accessible to anyone interested in working more effectively with children.

Play serves as language for a child and play therapy is a method of psychotherapy that utilizes play in an effort to help and understand a child (Kottman 1995; Landreth 1982). Children are more comfortable when they are allowed to use toys and play to express their thoughts, feelings, and problems. The techniques of play therapy which we use are based principally on the work of Dr. Terry Kottman (1993; 1995; Kottman & Schaefer 1993) an Adlerian play therapist. Her strategies at the most basic level apply four techniques: (1) tracking, (2) restating content, (3) reflecting feelings, and (4) encouraging. Tracking what a child says has no parallel in working with an adult (Kottman 1995). Tracking relates to narrating what a child is doing during the session (i.e., "You're picking that up. It is moving back and forth through the air"). While tracking a counselor should be very careful not to name the toy or object until the child does. Likewise, the counselor should not be naming the action the child is doing with the toy or object until the child does (i.e. Counselor: "You are picking that (puppet) up." Child: "It's a witch." Counselor: "You are picking up the witch (puppet). You are moving the witch." Child: "The witch is flying through the air.") In this way the counselor is not imposing his or her own version of reality on the child. Something as simple as calling a toy "he" or "she" should be avoided to allow the child time to give the object an identity and a purpose. Tracking what a child does gives the child verbal feedback on his/her actions. It lets the child know the counselor is at the child's level and helps to establish rapport.

Restating content does have a parallel when counseling with an adult. Restating content merely means saying what the child has just said in a slightly different way (i.e., the child says, "My baby is crying because it didn't get no supper!" The counselor says, "Your baby is crying because it is hungry.") When restating content, vocabulary level should be the same as the child's. Restating can be combined with tracking, but the counselor should be careful not to be talking all of the time. Restating content helps the child feel he or she has been heard, gives the child an opportunity to make a correction if the counselor has misunderstood, and is another step in building rapport with a child.

Reflecting feelings is yet another step in building a relationship with a child and again there is a parallel in counseling with adults. Similar to the technique used with adults, reflecting feelings with young children is more narrowly defined because young children usually only recognize and are able to verbalize five main feelings—sad, mad, glad (happy), scared, and guilty (Kottman, 1995). It is up to the counselor to ascertain what the child is feeling and to try to express it for the child (i.e., "You look sad when you talk about your grandmother." "You seem angry with people in the doll house.") If it is difficult to guess a feeling then a counselor can put himself/herself in the child's place by saying, "I'd be scared if . . . " or "I'd be happy if . . . ", to help elicit a verbalized feeling from the child. The one thing to avoid is saying something like, "Getting a present *makes you feel* happy." Saying "makes you feel" takes control away from the child and gives it to some external object or person. Reflecting feelings is an essential step in the process of allowing a child to recognize different emotions, the triggers to those emotions, and how to begin to cope with them.

Encouraging involves being able to value children for what they are as they come into the playroom. No outside elements should interfere, such as a previous reputation or an adult expectation of what the child *should* be. The adult needs to convey faith in and acceptance of the child and a positive belief in the child's abilities. Children pick up on this positive regard and begin to believe in themselves. Encouraging also involves recognizing not so much the deed that is done, but the effort that went into doing it. The product is not as important as noticing the joy and satisfaction in the process. If a child has difficulty in accomplishing something completely, the counselor can emphasize the good aspects of what was achieved. Some typical words of encouragement could be "You couldn't do that earlier, but now you did it!"; "You are really getting better at doing that!"; "You're really trying hard on that!"; "You figured that out for yourself!" Encouragement lets children hear that they have made progress.

Of course tracking, restating content, reflecting feelings, and encouraging are only the very, very basic techniques of play therapy. Other issues will arise such as setting limits, involving parents, using metaphors, etc. We encourage you to read some of the wealth of material available on play therapy. Our references include books by Terry Kottman, Garry Landreth, Violet Oaklander, and Virginia Axline.

TOYS

Toys are the tools of play intervention with children. All hospices should be able to utilize a small but diverse and appropriate collection of toys to assist children in acting out and resolving their feelings related to a significant death. A variety of suggested materials are presented here (Kottman 1995; Landreth 1982; Seager NHO Conference 1995). Your agency may choose to establish a fully equipped playroom or staff may keep a suitcase of relevant toys in their vehicle trunk. One may even choose to carry an "emergency" small plastic bag of appropriate toys in their purse or brief case. The cost can be quite minimal. Many of the items are available at garage sales or thrift stores. Several hospices have been able to fully equip playrooms solely through donations from their community of new and used toys. Another option when making a home visit is to utilize toys the child already owns.

Categories of Toys

In order for children to fully express their ideas and feelings, it is necessary to provide them with several categories of toys. There are five main categories. A toy room, satchel, or brief case should try to have some representation from each category.

Scary Toys: Children use these toys to deal with their fears, both real and imagined, present and past. This category includes such toys as snakes, roaches, rats, plastic monsters, dragons, dinosaurs, sharks, insects, and wolf, alligator and bear puppets, etc.

Family/Nurturing Toys: Children use these toys to explore family constellation and atmosphere, events that happen within the family unit, and for nurturing issues. This category includes doll houses, a doll family, people puppets, animal families, kitchenware, empty food containers, baby bottles, baby doll, doll clothes, stuffed toys, a child-size rocking chair, receiving blanket, iron, broom, etc.

Aggressive Toys: Children use these toys to express feelings of anger and fear, to learn to symbolically act out their aggression, to protect themselves from threats, and to explore issues of power, control and trust. Such toys could include a punching bag, toy guns, plastic or rubber knives, handcuffs, a plastic shield, tools for pounding such as a hammer or mallet, toy soldiers, small pillows for a pillow fight, foam rubber bats, etc.

Expressive Toys: Children use these to explore family relationships, express feelings, symbolically work out problems and solutions, and to express creativity. This category of toys includes crayons, scissors, markers, watercolors, tempura, scotch tape, pipe cleaners, egg cartons, newsprint, glue, play dough, an easel, etc.

Pretend/Fantasy Toys: Children use these toys to explore different roles, express hidden feelings, practice alternative behaviors, pretend to be someone else, and use fantasy to explore relationships and communicate important ideas metaphorically. These toys include masks, hats, jewelry, purses, disguises, a telephone, a doctor kit, blocks, magic wands, puppets, puppet theater, sand box (or dishpan full of rice or beans), a white sheet, zoo and farm animals, and building materials, etc. Pretend/Fantasy toys should not have a preconceived identity with television shows, movies, etc., so that children can impose their own ideas and identities on the toys.

Toys for the Ideal Playroom

A small sandbox or dishpan full of rice or dry beans, a doctor kit, a white sheet, telephone, doll house and furniture, an assortment of cars and trucks, Gumby, small plastic animals (both zoo and farm animals), toy stove and dishes, easel and paint, markers, crayons, finger paints, glue, scotch tape, bendable figures, hats, soft dart gun, machine gun, toy soldiers, handcuffs, empty cans and food boxes, hand puppets, mask, rubber balls, egg cartons, pipe cleaners, table, chairs, doll bed, airplane, doll clothes, paper dolls, iron, broom, mop, rags, stuffed animals, old hats, purse, magic wand or other "wishing" toy, the Ungame, the Nurturing Game, and running water, if possible. Toys in a playroom should be arranged by category, in full view, and easily accessible.

Toys for a Large Portable Suitcase

Crayons and washable felt tip markers, newsprint, blunt scissors, plastic baby bottle, Gumby, rubber knife, doll, play dough, small plain mask, dart gun, toy soldiers, empty can, play dishes, small cars or trucks, hand puppets, bendable doll family and portable doll house, rubber ball, glue, scotch tape, egg carton, pipe cleaners, telephone, handcuffs, doctor kit, magic wand or other small "wishing" toy.

Toys for a Small Satchel

Crayons, markers, 8 × 10 pad of plain paper, small blunt scissors, scotch tape, small baby and baby bottle, family of people or animal figures, small dinosaur or monster figures, soft dart gun, rubber knife, small can of play dough, a "scary" puppet, fantasy or friendly puppet, small cars or trucks, dark glasses, pipe cleaners, plastic toy soldiers, stickers or colorforms.

Toys for a Small Plastic Bag

Crayons, small pad of paper, micro cars, tiny family of people or animal figures or finger puppets, deck of cards, small plastic monsters or dinosaurs, "magic" ring, silly putty, dark glasses, stickers, pen (to write on fingers) 3 or 4 plastic soldiers.

HANDS-ON INTERVENTION STRATEGIES
(based on Seager, NHO Conference 1995)

The goal of utilizing toys, art, music, and other materials with children is to allow them to express and deal with their feelings effectively. These strategies are designed to be low cost and portable.

To work with the child, seek a place that is private or neutral. Any location can be used from an established toy room to the kitchen table with others out of the room, the child's room, an empty classroom or office at school, a fast food place, a park, the front steps with no one around, even the back seat of a car.

With Paper and Crayons

Have the child draw for you. Use large white paper and a medium to large box of crayons (must include black, red and yellow).

If the child is reluctant it often helps if you make a picture but on your own paper. Perhaps allow the child to direct what you should draw and you direct what they should draw.

1. Draw me a picture of the family before . . . (Dad got sick, Mom died, etc.). Then draw me a picture of the family now. Lastly, draw a picture of how the family will be a year from now. Make everyone in the picture doing something.

Moderate the energy level and concentration ability of the child. They may not be able to do all three pictures in one session.

2. Draw me a picture of how you feel about . . . /how you felt when . . . (Sister died, you went to the hospital to see Grandma, etc.)
3. Draw anger/sadness/love, etc.
4. Draw a picture of_____in Heaven. (If concurrent with family belief system.)
5. Draw a picture of a favorite activity with . . . (Dad, Sis, etc.)
6. Draw a picture of what you miss the most about . . . (Grandpa, etc.)

Ask questions about the pictures which elicit information and avoid generating yes/no, one-word answers. For example, don't ask "Is that a house?" or "What is that?"

Never guess about a drawing. The correct wording is "Please tell me about it." You may narrate the drawing process without adding definition ("You are making a big circle. It is a red circle. Now you are making the center black.")

When the picture is complete and you are discussing it, try "You have made the little girl all in yellow. How does she feel about that?", or, "I see you have used a lot of purple. Can you tell me why you chose that color today?" Ask how the people in the picture feel. "What were they doing before this time?" "What will she be doing tonight?" "I wonder what that little boy is thinking?"

Colors chosen, details of anatomy (no arms, for example), relative positioning and sizes of persons, and inclusion or exclusion in the picture of significant persons all give ideas of how the child feels about things.

Never criticize anything the child draws. For example, don't say "You have drawn your brother being blown up by tanks. That is not a nice thing to do."

7. Fold the paper into boats which can be decorated or identified as individuals who have a relationship (even a "family" of boats) or utilized as tools for the child to express feelings such as anger, escape, peril, etc.

Easily Accessible Things to Do

Children will not sit down quietly and discuss their feelings. To establish a relationship with a child in a patient/family, give the child some undivided attention. This doesn't always have to be a long time; even twenty minutes can be helpful. Use materials such as pipe cleaners, modeling clay/play dough, Legos. Outside you can use bubbles, toss a ball, etc. Allow the child to play or fiddle with the activity while you talk. You may also want to participate.

> Talk about safe, neutral things (school, favorite TV show) and bring up other issues only as you feel the child is receptive. Watch for signs such as suddenly stopping the activity, non sequiturs, or changing the subject. This may indicate that the topic is threatening to the child. Above all, developing your rapport with the child is more important than getting information. Developing trust is essential.

Worksheets and More

There are various commercial activity sheets which can be used with youth. Some of them are easy to construct yourself. For example:

1. Have the child draw how they feel (i.e. "happy, sad, mad," etc.) on an empty outline of a face. Sometimes it is good if the therapist also draws how they feel. Use this as a starting point. "You have drawn an angry face today. Can you tell me why you are angry?"
2. Make a mood barometer. Draw a tall rectangle with a bulb at the bottom. Mark it with different feeling states from really down at the bottom to great at the top. Have the child mark the place on the barometer that reflects how he/she feels today. Use vocabulary that will relate to the child ("sad, blue, depressed, lonely, pretty good, terrific, awesome," etc.).
3. (With older kids.) Make a time line. Put in significant events. Put in hopes for the future. Decorate it with drawings or cut out pictures from magazines.
4. Make paper dolls. Draw or trace outlines of people or animals (such as dinosaurs) on plain paper and have the child color them. Glue them on cardboard, cut them out and play with them. Try to have available characters which relate to the child's situation (i.e., grandparent dolls, doctor and nurse dolls, family of dolls, etc.).

Making a Book

Assist the child or children to make a book about hospice coming to see the patient, treatment, the death/funeral experience, and/or how they feel.

You may want to use *Homemade Books To Help Kids Cope* by Robert Ziegler, M.D. (see Appendix 2) as a guide. The child can dictate to you or a volunteer, or use a computer or tape recorder for the text. Volunteers may be able to transcribe. Have the child do the illustrations and/or use photographs.

With a Tape Recorder

1. Use the tape recorder to say things someone else should say. ("If Mom was here, what would she say to you?")
2. Use the tape recorder (name it: "This is Jeffy. This is how Jeffy would/does feel") to say things the child wants to say but feels he shouldn't. ("I hate Dad being sick all the time. I wish he would just die and go away.")
3. Use the tape recorder to leave messages for others (i.e., with a terminal child).

Always ask the child if you may keep or copy the tape. Give it to them if they want it or erase it altogether if they ask. Promise not to let Mom/Dad/significant adult hear it without the child's permission.

Games and Cards

1. Play a game such as The Nurturing Game or an old favorite such as Chutes and Ladders. Use the game to establish rapport or to create a safe place for the child to talk with you.
2. Use playing cards the same way or allow the child to play creatively with them, making up games, assigning persons to the face cards, etc. ("Which card would be you? Which one would be Mom? What does the "you" card have to say to the "Mom" card?")

Making Believe

1. Empty Chair
   Pretend someone who is not present or is deceased is sitting in an empty chair. Assist the child in talking with this person. For example, "If Grandpa was sitting here, what would he say to you?" "What if Mom was sitting here? What do you want to say to her?"
2. Imaginary Friend
   Utilize the concept of an imaginary friend to vocalize things the child has trouble owning or saying, or perhaps needs to hear from a

"safe" source. "If you had an imaginary friend here with us, what would they do? say? Can you show me?"

3. Someone Else

Ask the child, "If you could be someone else, who/what would you be? What would you do?" The therapist often needs to join in the play. Ask the child who you should be and what you should do.

4. Dress Up

Use old clothing, costumes, hats, disguises, costume jewelry, purses, shoes, etc., to take on different roles and "act out" feelings/concerns.

5. Magic

A magic wand (which is easy to construct from doweling and glitter, etc.), Aladdin's Lamp, or "magic ring" (any large gaudy ring from a thrift shop) and other such materials all provide opportunities for the child to access hope, the future, and identify personal goals. This is a very successful and powerful intervention technique.

6. Dream Catchers

Dream Catchers can be constructed from commercial kits or inexpensive materials at any craft shop. Allow the child to choose colors and specific things to attach such as beads, feathers, pictures, mementos. Empower the dream catcher to thwart nightmares or capture happy memories.

Puppets

Use all kinds of puppets to act out stories and feelings–store-bought, home made, full hand puppets, finger puppets, etc. Even drawing faces on a child's fingers.

Spirit Puppets

Families of many different religious traditions often explain death in terms of a spirit leaving the body and going to heaven, etc. This is a very difficult concept for young children. Using a glove to demonstrate this (the hand and fingers are the spirit, the glove the body, which cannot move without the spirit) is sometimes helpful. Women's dress gloves are often available at thrift shops and faces, etc., can be drawn on them with markers. A volunteer could easily stitch up simple "ghost" puppets of skin-colored cloth and these can also be drawn on with markers. The craft activity can make the whole subject less frightening and more accessible to the children. (Let them keep the puppets/gloves.)

Bibliotherapy

There are many excellent books to read with youth and to discuss afterwards, covering all topics of illness, death and dying, and grief, etc. Books can be used to bring up certain topics or address specific issues (See Appendix 2).

Music

Music is a wonderfully creative tool to work with persons of all ages. Music can be used to set a mood, create calm, and to express feelings. Music can resurrect memories. With children, pre-written music (recorded or in books) can be used as well as opportunities to create their own songs and music. Skill levels of the child and the adult are not important.

Newsletter (Appendix 1)

Help the children write and produce a weekly or monthly newsletter about themselves or, preferably, the whole family. It can be hand written, typed or done on a computer, even filmed with videotape. A staff person or a volunteer could possibly type it for them. Add on some art work or clip art.

Suggestions for content:

> Interview the hospice nurse/volunteer/social worker/homemaker-home health aide, etc.
> Interview family members
> Write about the medications
> Write about the funeral
> Write about a special memory or remembered funny story

THINGS TO REMEMBER IN WORKING WITH CHILDREN

Never force an activity or a conversation. When the child is tired or threatened, just let him/her play without an agenda or terminate the session. Be prepared to be flexible. For example, a child may refuse to draw but be willing to dump out the crayons and play with them as persons and use the empty box as their house. By noting the play, colors he/she chooses to play different persons, etc., a dialogue can begin.

Explain confidentiality to the child and to the parents/significant adults. To the child, say something like, "I won't tell your parents anything which you don't want them to know, unless I feel that there is a chance you or someone could be injured." To the significant adults, explain that the child needs the security of knowing they will not be punished for having "bad" or "wrong" feelings and won't be put into the situation where something which might "hurt" another's feelings would be revealed to that person.

In communicating with parents/significant adults, be aware of their concerns and that they may be dealing with issues similar to those of the child. In some situations, it is wiser to share summaries of content, rather than many specifics. The adults may be less comprehending of the developmental status of the child and the need of the child to act out both positive and negative feelings through their activities. Sometimes significant adults can be inclined to be more judgmental of the child than the therapist or misinterpret the child's need to express feelings from the child having "wrong" feelings. As an example, say "Missy feels left out sometimes when her brother Mark is especially sick/having pain/getting chemotherapy," rather than saying, "Missy is sometimes jealous of Mark and in play pretends she also has a 'bad' disease so that she gets the toys and attention."

CONCLUSION

Allowing children to express and deal with their feelings concerning the death of a significant person in a safe and non-judgmental atmosphere can prevent unresolved grief later in adult life. Youth are as vital a part of hospice patient/families as adults, regardless of whether they are the patient, sibling, children, grandchildren or special friend. This paper provides trained hospice human service professionals the information they need to effectively understand and intervene with children grieving a death or impending death.

REFERENCES

Axline, Virginia (1964). *Dibs in search of self.* New York: Ballantine Books.

Corr, Charles (1995). Children's understandings of death-striving to understand death. *Children Mourning, Mourning Children,* Kenneth Doka (editor). Washington, D.C.: Hospice Foundation of America.

Grollman, E. (1990). *Talking about death (a dialogue between parent and child).* Boston, MA: Beacon Press.

Grollman, E. (1995). NHO conference keynote speech. San Francisco, CA.

Kottman, T. (1993). Adlerian play therapy workshop material. Waterloo, Iowa: Cedar Valley Hospice.

Kottman, T. (1995). *Partners in play.* Alexandria, VA: American Counseling Association.

Kottman, T. and Schaefer, C., editors (1993). *Play therapy in action: A casebook for practitioners.* Northvale, NJ: Jason Aronson Inc.

Landreth, Garry, ed. (1982). *Play therapy, dynamics of the process of counseling with children.* Springfield, IL: Charles C. Thomas.

Oaklander, Violet (1988). *Windows to our children.* Highland, New York: Gestalt Journal Press.

Papenbrock, P. and Voss, Robert (1988). *Children's grief–how to help the child whose parent has died.* Redmond, WA: Mecic Publishing Company.

Schaefer, Dan and Lyons, Christine (1993). *How do we tell the children?* New York: New Market Press.

Seager, Kathleen Muleady (1995) NHO conference presentation, "Meeting the Needs of Kids in Patient/Families–Not Just Playing Around." San Francisco, CA.

Spencer, Susan C. (1995) NHO conference presentation, "Meeting the Needs of Kids in Patient/Families–Not Just Playing Around." San Francisco, CA.

APPENDIX 1. The Smith Family Newsletter

EDITED BY JAKE AND SARAH SMITH   JULY, 1995

DAD GETS HOSPITAL BED
By Sarah Smith
Today Dad got a new bed from
Hospice. It is in the living
room. It goes up and down by
itself. I like Dad in the
living room.

[clip art here]

[diagram of bed here]

AUNT JANNEY COMES TO
VISIT
By Jake Smith
Dad's sister Aunt Janney is
here from Florida. She
brought Jake and Sarah T-
shirts with alligators on
them. They are awesome.

Aunt Janney cried a lot the
first time she saw Dad. We
told her it was OK to cry.
Aunt Janney says "I am
happy to be here but I am sad Dad
is so sick."

APPENDIX 1 (continued)

PICTURE BY JAKE

KATIE KOALA IS KOOL
By Sarah Smith
Katie Koala came to see us again.
She brought us stickers but no
more bears. She even hugged Mom!

MARY LOU THE NURSE
By Jake Smith

Mary Lou is Dad's nurse. She
has one kid but she is grown
up. Mary Lou brings Dad
medicine to take away the
pain. Mary Lou likes horses.

A POEM BY SARAH
xxxxxxxxxxxxxxxxx
xxxxxxxxxxxxxxxxx
etc.

[more clip art here]

APPENDIX 2
BIBLIOTHERAPY AND PROFESSIONAL RESOURCES

Preschool–Kindergarten

Buscaglia, L. (1982). *The Fall of Freddie the Leaf.* New Jersey: Charles B.
   Slack. *The story of a leaf named Freddie and his life through the
   changing seasons.*
Clifton, L. & Grifalconi, A. (1988). *Everett Anderson's Goodbye.* New
   York: Henry Holt. *A little boy struggles through the five stages of grief
   as he tries to come to grips with the death of his father.*
Mellonie, B. & Ingpen, R. (1983). *Lifetimes: The Beautiful Way to Explain
   Death to Children.* New York: Bantam Books. *A simply written book
   with illustrations that helps explain death as part of the natural cycle of
   all living things.*
Klicker, R. (1988). *Kolie and the Funeral.* Buffalo, NY: Thanos Institute.
   *Ten page story/coloring book using words and pictures to explain death
   and funerals to young children.*
Rogers, F. (1988). *When a Pet Dies.* New York: Putnam. *Excellent color
   photographs help children explore and understand emotions, fears, and
   concerns when a pet dies.*

Sanford, D. (1986). *It Must Hurt a Lot.* Portland, OR: Multnomah Press. *After a boy's dog is killed, he learns to express his emotions and to grow through his memories and grief.*

Sanford, D. (1988). *In Our Neighborhood, David Has AIDS.* Oregon: Multnomah Press. *David is a hemophiliac who has contracted AIDS from a blood transfusion. Through a friendship and the wisdom of his grandmother, David is able to face his approaching death.*

Varley, S. (1984). *Badger's Parting Gifts.* New York: Mulberry Books. *All the woodland creatures–Mole, Frog, Fox, and Rabbit–love old Badger, who is their confidante, advisor, and friend. When he dies, they are overwhelmed by their loss. Then, they begin to remember.*

Wilhelm, H. (1985). *I'll Always Love You.* New York: Crown Publishers, Inc. *A little boy deals with the death of "the best dog in the whole world."*

Primary (1st–5th)

Boulden, Jim & Brett (1992). *Uncle Jerry Has AIDS.* California: Boulden Publishing. *Noncontroversial, highly effective material for processing attitudes and emotions held by children in the first to fifth grades.*

Bunting, E. (1982). *The Happy Funeral.* New York: Harper & Row. *Laura and her family attend her grandfather's funeral and participate in Chinese mourning rituals. Describes Chinese funeral customs.*

Cohn, J. (1987). *I Had a Friend Named Peter.* New York: Wm. Morrow. *Beth's friend, Peter, is killed by a car. Her parents and teacher sensitively answer questions.*

Clifford, E. (1985). *The Remembering Box.* Boston, MA: Houghton, Mifflin. *Nine-year-old Joshua spent every Sabbath with his Grandma learning about the old country, her family, and her life through her remembering box. This helped Joshua to understand and accept his Grandma's death and the various Jewish rituals that were an important part of her life.*

Donnelly, E. (1981). *So Long, Grandpa.* New York: Crown. *Michael at 10 witnesses the deterioration and eventual death from cancer of his grandfather. Portrays Michael's reactions. The grandfather prepares the boy by taking him to the funeral of a friend.*

Gould, D. (1987). *Grandpa's Slide Show.* New York: Lothrop, Lee, and Shepard. *Grandpa's slide shows are a regular event during his grandchildren's visits until he becomes very ill, is hospitalized, and dies. Describes young children's grief behavior and their participation in the funeral. That evening Mom helps with the slide show which has great meaning for Grandma, too.*

APPENDIX 2 (continued)

Miles, M. (1971). *Annie and the Old One*. Boston, MA: Atlantic-Little, Brown. *Annie, a Navajo Indian girl, tries to prevent her grandmother's death by undoing the rug she is weaving. Grandmother helps her understand dying in the context of life-cycle rhythms.*

O'Toole, D. (1988). *Aarvy Aardvark Finds Hope*. Burnsville, NC: Celo Press. *An illustrated read-aloud story of the pain and sadness of loss and the hope of grief recovery.*

Paterson, K. (1977). *Bridge to Terabithia*. New York: Crowell. *Jesse and Leslie have their own special, secret meeting place in the woods, which they call "Terabithia." The magic of their play is disrupted when one of them is killed in an accident on the way to visit Terabithia alone. The remaining child learns to deal with the grief and initiate new relationships.*

Prestine, Joan Singleton (1993). *Someone Special Died*. Carthage, IL: Fearon Teacher Aids. *Excellent accompanying book to a practical resource guide for teachers. A little girl goes through the stages of grief after "someone special" in her life dies. (See Adult Bib.)*

Rylant, Cynthia (1992). *Missing May*. New York: Dell Publishing. *Since Summer was six years old, she has lived with dear Aunt May and Uncle Ob. Now, six years later, May has died. Summer, who misses May with all her might, is afraid something will happen to Ob. Together they set off on a search for some sign of May to ease their sorrow and give them strength.*

Smith, D. B. (1973). *A Taste of Blackberries*. New York: Scholastic. *The story of the death of Jamie, the narrator's best friend, as a result of an allergic reaction to a bee sting and the narrator's reflections on this unexpected event.*

Taha, K. (1986). *A Gift for Tia Rosa*. New York: Bantam Books. *Tia Rosa is teaching Carmela how to knit and everyday the two friends work on their special projects together. Carmela is sure that Tia Rosa will get well, but one day she runs home to find her friend gone and comes up with her own special tribute.*

Wilson, J. M. (1990). *Robin On His Own*. New York: Scholastic. *A black boy whose family is in transition tries to come to terms with the death of his mother. The book gives fresh dimensions to the idea of family and a boy's courage in learning when to hold on and when to let go.*

White, E. B. (1952). *Charlotte's Web*. New York: Harper. *When Charlotte, a spider, dies, her friends Wilbur, a pig, and Templeton, a rat, grieve and remember the special things about her. The birth of Charlotte's children brings some comfort.*

Middle–High School (6th-12th)

Armstrong, W. H. (1969). *Sounder.* New York: Harper & Row. *The coming-of-age story of a young black boy in turn-of-the-century rural South. How he deals with the crippling of his beloved hound, Sounder, and the imprisonment of his father, and the ultimate deaths of both form the focus of the story.*

Blume, Judy (1981). *Tiger Eyes.* New York: Dell Publishing. *Teenager Davey's father is murdered in a hold-up and she and her family have moved to New Mexico to recover. Lonely Davey meets the mysterious Wolf, and only he understands the rage and fear that she feels. Slowly, Davey learns to get on with her life.*

Fleischman, P. (1986). *Rear-View Mirror.* New York: Harper & Row. *After visiting her father for the first time, Olivia must deal with his sudden death: only then does she realize her own self worth.*

Hermes, P. (1982). *You Shouldn't Have to Say Goodbye.* New York: Scholastic. *From the moment 13 year old Sarah Morrow hugs her mother one dreary afternoon, it's clear that something is wrong. Days later Sarah's mom checks into the hospital and is diagnosed with inoperable cancer. Unwilling to accept the news, Sarah throws herself into gymnastics practice and with the help of her friend struggles to believe that everything will be okay. As Sarah, her mom, and her dad confront what they are about to lose, each finds real happiness in the time that is left.*

Holland, I. (1989). *Of Love and Death and Other Journeys.* Greenwich, CT: Fawcett. *As Meg's mother dies of cancer, Meg's childhood dies too. Meg can accept a changed future when she is finally able to grieve.*

Krementz, Jill (1991). *How it Feels When a Parent Dies,* New York: Alfred Knopf. *Eighteen children from seven to sixteen speak openly of their experience.*

Mazer, N. (1987) *After the Rain.* New York: Morrow. *The bittersweet experience of a 15-year-old girl's relationship with her dying grandfather.*

Sanders, D. (1990). *Clover.* New York: Ballantine Books. *Clover, a 10 year old black girl from a small town in South Carolina, chronicles her bewildering, but gradually deepening relationship with her white stepmother following her father's tragic death only hours after the marriage.*

Adult

Fitzgerald, Helen (1992). *The Grieving Child* (A Parent's Guide). New York: Fireside. *Practical guide for any parent who wishes to help a child cope with grief.*

APPENDIX 2 (continued)

Kubler-Ross, Elisabeth (1983). *On Children and Death.* New York: Mac-Millan Publishing Co. *How children and their parents can and do cope with death.*

Grollman, Earl (1990). *Talking About Death: A Dialogue Between Parent and Child.* Boston: Beacon Press. *Simple straightforward language used to tell the story of a loved one's death. Includes illustrations and parent's guide.*

Linn, E. (1990). *150 Facts About Grieving Children.* Incline Village, NV: Publisher's Mark. *Important information to help caring adults recognize possible characteristics of children dealing with any type of grief.*

Schaefer, Dan & Lyons, Christine (1993). *How Do We Tell the Children?* New York: Newmarket Press. *A step-by-step guide for helping children two to teen cope when someone dies.*

Wolfelt, A. (1983). *Helping Children Cope with Grief.* Muncie, IN: Accelerated Development.

Resources for Professionals

Eth, Spencer & Mitchell, Jeffrey (1989). *Trauma in the Lives of Children, Alameda, CA: Hunter House Inc. Crisis and stress management techniques for counselors and other professionals.*

Kottman, Terry (1995). *Partners in Play,* Alexandria, VA: American Counseling Association. *Step-by-step instructions on how to integrate the concepts and techniques of Adlerian Psychology in the practice of play therapy.*

Kottman, Terry & Schaefer, Charles (1993). *Play Therapy in Action: A Casebook for Practitioners.* Northvale, NJ: Jason Aronson, Inc. *Concrete applications of play therapy by seasoned clinicians from various theoretical backgrounds.*

Landreth, Gary L. (1982). *Play Therapy* (Dynamics of the Process of Counseling with Children). Springfield, IL: Charles C. Thomas.

Morgan, John D. (1990). *The Dying and the Bereaved Teenager.* The Charles Press, Publishers, Inc., Philadelphia, PA. *Protocols schools can adopt or adapt to help young people cope.*

Nemiroff, Marc & Annunziata, Jane (1990). *A Child's First Book About Play Therapy.* Washington, D.C.: American Psychological Association. *A book to be read to young children age 4 to 7 by a parent or therapist.*

Pardeck, John & Pardeck, Jean, editors (1993). *Bibliotherapy, A Clinical Approach for Helping Children.* USA: Gordon and Breach Science Publishers.

Prestine, Joan Singleton (1993). *Helping Children Cope With Death* (A Practical Resource Guide For "Someone Special Died"). Carthage, IL: Fearon Teacher Aids. *Excellent Preschool–grade 3 guide on communicating with children about death. Many book and activity suggestions.*

Webb, N. B. (1991). *Play Therapy With Children in Crisis.* New York: The Guilford Press. *A casebook illustrating a variety of play therapy techniques.*

Wolfelt, Alan (1983). *Helping Children Cope With Grief.* Muncie, IN: Accelerated Development, Inc. *A handbook for parents, teachers, and counselors.*

Ziegler, Robert G. (1992). *Homemade Books to Help Kids Cope.* New York: Magination Press. *An easy-to-learn technique for parents and professionals on how to create personalized books for and with children.*

Workbooks for Children

Boulden, Jim & Boulden, Brett (1992). *Uncle Jerry Has AIDS.* Weaverville, CA: Boulden Publishing. *An activity book to help young children deal with questions about AIDS.*

Boulden, Jim & Boulden, Joan (1994). *Goodbye Forever.* Weaverville, CA: Boulden Publishing. *Bereavement activity book for children kindergarten through second grade.*

Boulden, Jim & Boulden, Joan (1992). *Saying Goodbye.* Weaverville, CA: Boulden Publishing. *Bereavement activity book for children.*

Deaton, Wendy (1994). *Someone I Love Died.* Alameda, CA: Hunter House, Inc. *A child's workbook about loss and grieving. Comes with therapist guide and reproducible worksheets.*

Grollman, Earl A. (1987). *A Scrapbook of Memories.* Batesville, IN: Batesville Management Services. *A scrapbook to be completed by a child who has had a loved one die.*

Levine, Jennifer (1992). *Forever In My Heart.* Burnsville, NC: Mountain Rainbow Publications. *A story to help children participate in life as a parent dies.*

Media Resources

Blackberries in the Dark. 16 mm film–Walt Disney Films. 1/2" VHS video–Coronet Centron. *The touching story of nine-year-old Austin and his grandmother and their personal struggle to come to terms with the recent death of Austin's grandfather.*

Can't Live With 'Em. 1/2" VHS video–Direct Cinema. *The Degrassi High kids are back at school in a one-hour special. Wheels struggles with grief and guilt when his parents are killed in a car accident.*

APPENDIX 2 (continued)

Growing Old. 16 mm film–Encyclopedia Britannica. *Explores the nature of people's reactions to aging and death.*

It Must Hurt A Lot. VHS video, Franciscan Communications. *The story of young Joshua and the accidental death of his beloved pet Muffin.*

Ramona: Goodbye, Hello. 16mm film–Churchill Films. *The death of Picky-Picky, the family's pet cat, brings Ramona and Beezus closer together.*

Saying Good-bye. VHS video–Aquarius Productions, Inc. *Several different teens talk about their experiences before and after the death of a parent or sibling. Two versions of the tape–one for teens, one for adults.*

A Tangled Web. 1/2" VHS video–Direct Cinema. *Still struggling to cope with his parents' death, Wheels is acting out in school and at home. After he has a confrontation with his grandmother, she asks him to leave.*

Techniques of Play Therapy. VHS video–Guilford Publications, Inc. *Nancy Boyd Webb, a noted authority on play therapy, describes and demonstrates techniques.*

Tenth Good Thing About Barney. 16 mm film–AIMS. *When Barney the cat died, his family gave him a funeral in their backyard and the young boy was brokenhearted. The mother suggested he think of ten good things about Barney.*

We're Almost Home Now. VHS video–Aquarius Productions, Inc. *A comprehensive look at Elisabeth Kubler-Ross's concept of the grieving process through her revolutionary work with dying children. Includes art techniques that she uses with children.*

What About Me? VHS video–Film Ideas, Inc. *Eleven children discuss their experiences of grief due to the death or chronic illness of a sibling or parent.*

What Do I Tell My Children? VHS video–Aquarius Productions, Inc. NHO "Film of the Year" award. *An outstanding resource for families and professionals who are helping children to cope with the death of a loved one.*

Transcending a Devastating Loss:
The Life Attitude of Mothers
Who Have Experienced the Death
of Their Only Child

Kay Talbot

SUMMARY. This study measured 80 mothers' attitudes about life five or more years after the death of their only child (mean = nine years). Participants completed the Life Attitude Profile-Revised. The five highest and five lowest scoring mothers were interviewed in depth. Discriminant analysis of participant questionnaires revealed that 86% of participants were correctly classified by seven variables as survivors (reinvestors in life) or as remaining in a state of perpetual bereavement. Four of these variables accounted for 39% of the variance in participants' life attitude scores. Interview and questionnaire findings suggest motherhood becomes an integral part of the self and in order to survive after the death of an only child it is necessary not to relinquish this construct. A positive life attitude was

Kay Talbot, PhD, is a grief counselor and consultant in private practice in Vallejo, CA. Her daughter and only child, Leah Talbot, died in 1982 at the age of nine.

Address correspondence to: Kay Talbot, PhD, 180 Wildflower Avenue, Vallejo, CA 94591 (e-mail: KayTalbot@aol.com).

My enduring gratitude and admiration to the participants in this study who courageously shared both their happy memories of motherhood and their painful experiences of bereavement.

[Haworth co-indexing entry note]: "Transcending a Devastating Loss: The Life Attitude of Mothers Who Have Experienced the Death of Their Only Child." Talbot, Kay. Co-published simultaneously in *The Hospice Journal* (The Haworth Press, Inc.) Vol. 11, No. 4, 1996, pp. 67-82: and: *Bereavement: Client Adaptation and Hospice Services* (ed: Donna Lind Infeld, and Nadine Reimer Penner) The Haworth Press, Inc., 1996, pp. 67-82. Single or multiple copies of this article are available for a fee from The Haworth Document Delivery Service [1-800-342-9678, 9:00 a.m. - 5:00 p.m. (EST). E-mail address: getinfo@haworth.com].

found to be an important indicator of adaptation to this unique form of bereavement. *[Article copies available for a fee from The Haworth Document Delivery Service: 1-800-342-9678. E-mail address: getinfo@ haworth.com]*

INTRODUCTION

Bereavement researchers have concluded that the phenomenon of parental bereavement is the most difficult form of bereavement (Cleiren, 1993; Knapp, 1986; Osterweis, Solomon, and Green, 1984; Rando, 1986; Sanders, 1979-80, 1989). This is because the loss is multifaceted. Parents lose not only their unique relationship with a valued and loved child, they lose the part of themselves that child represents. They lose the future they and the child would otherwise have created together. They lose the immortality of being survived by the child and the child's descendants. And they lose their false illusions about the degree of control they have over life (Edelstein, 1984).

The emotional, cognitive, physical, social, and spiritual changes which result from the loss of a child work together to confront bereaved parents with a heightened responsibility for a new existence. The additional loss of the role of parent which accompanies the death of an only child adds to this existential crisis. Virtually every aspect of their lives is irrevocably altered. In studying the process of role exit, Ebaugh (1988) found that role residual was common to all who exited a role, voluntarily or not. Role residual is "the identification that an individual maintains with a prior role such that the individual experiences certain aspects of the role after he or she has in fact exited from it" (Ebaugh, 1988, p. 173). Further, "the more personal involvement and commitment an individual had in a former role, that is, the more self-identity was equated with role definitions, the more role residual tended to manifest itself after the exit" (p. 178). While bereaved mothers were not included in Ebaugh's study, I postulated that for many bereaved mothers the role of motherhood is highly correlated with self-identity and for these mothers, the loss of their role as a mother intensifies the identity conflict that is already made extant by the loss of the part of themselves that the child signified. I hypothesized that mothers who have survived the death of their only child to reinvest in life again—a life that has goals, hope, trust, and meaning—will have found ways to successfully incorporate "mothering" into their new lives.

METHOD

To measure life attitude, I used the Life Attitude Profile-Revised (LAP-R) (Reker & Peacock, 1981). The LAP-R contains six scales which measure (1) life purpose; (2) life coherence; (3) life control; (4) death acceptance; (5) existential vacuum; and (6) goal seeking. Scores from the six LAP-R scales were used to calculate a Life Attitude Balance Index (LABI) which takes into account both the degree to which meaning and purpose in life have been discovered and the motivation to find meaning and purpose (Reker, 1992). I reasoned that the range of possible LABI scores provided by the LAP-R instrument could represent a bereavement continuum, with those scoring low representing a state of perpetual bereavement and those scoring high representing survival. In order to understand the experience of survival, I also found it necessary to understand the experience of not surviving, of remaining perpetually bereaved after the death of an only child.

I recruited participants through the mailing list of Alive Alone, Inc. (Bevington, 1993) which provides a newsletter and networking opportunities for bereaved parents with no surviving children. Eighty mothers who met the study criteria completed the LAP-R, the Perceived Well-Being Index (PWB-R) (Reker & Wong, 1984), and a lengthy questionnaire containing demographic information and variables related to grief resolution. I performed the following statistical analysis of responses to the questionnaire: correlation, discriminant, multiple regression, and chi square analysis.

LABI scores for the 80 participants ranged from -8 (lowest) to 162 (highest), which compares to a total possible range of -80 (lowest) to 208 (highest). The distribution of participant scores approximated a normal curve, with a mean of 84.6 and standard deviation of 38.62. As expected, participants' LABI scores were somewhat negatively skewed from those of the normative sample which consisted of 491 women (mean = 94.1, standard deviation = 29.98; $p < .01$) [Reker, 1992, p. 46]. The PWB-R scores of the participants correlated highly with LABI scores ($r = .7691$; $p < .0005$). Accordingly, I determined it was not necessary to use this second instrument to identify women to interview. I selected an interview sample of ten participants to represent both ends of the conceptualized continuum: five with the highest and five with the lowest LABI scores.

I conducted tape recorded interviews which lasted from 2-1/2 to 5-1/2 hours in the participants' homes. I began each interview with the same question: "What do I need to know in order to understand what it has been like for you to survive the death of your only child?" Follow-up probes were used as necessary; however, the form of the interviews was dynamic and conversational, with the answers given to my questions continually informing the evolving conversation. I shared my own bereavement experience with the participants as seemed appropriate during our conversations. However, my aim was to encourage the participants' speaking rather than my own, and I carefully chose the points at which I interrupted them since doing so would have the potential of changing the topic of discussion.[1] The transcribed, verbatim interview texts were subjected to a phenomenological content analysis (Giorgi, 1975; Hycner, 1985).

PARTICIPANT CHARACTERISTICS

The 80 participants live in 32 different states, and are predominantly white (94%), married (66%), and college graduates (51%). Fifty-six percent work full-time outside their homes. Of those who work either full or part-time, 21% started working after the death of their child. Forty-five percent of the women have an annual family income of $50,000 or more. Sixty-three percent are involved in some type of volunteer activity for their church, bereavement group, local charities, local schools, or other community service organizations. Of these women, 39% began volunteering after the death of their child. Three women stopped volunteering after the death of their child.

All but three of the women reported a religious affiliation, predominantly Protestant. Half of the women said they had changed either their religious affiliation or their spiritual beliefs since their child's death.

These 80 women had been bereaved an average of nine years, with 68% bereaved from five to 13 years. Seventy-seven percent of the children who died were between the ages of 14 and 21, and 73% of the deaths were accidental, predominantly automobile-related.

RESULTS

Seven variables from the Participant Questionnaire correlated strongly with the participants' LABI scores and were selected as the independent variables for discriminant analysis. These seven variables, with corresponding discriminant function coefficients shown in brackets, were:

1. How helpful participants felt their friends were. [.54276]
2. Participants' involvement in volunteer activities. [.44579]

---

1. At the end of the interview, several mothers said they would never have shared certain aspects of their experience if I had not been a bereaved mother also.

3. Participants' level of education. [− .15753]
4. Amount of time elapsed between when the participant first realized the child might die and the child's death. [.24877]
5. Annual family income level. [.46705]
6. How helpful participants felt their religious or spiritual beliefs were. [.05863]
7. How frequently participants discussed their grief with others. [.41836]

Discriminant analysis showed that 86% of the women were correctly classified by these seven independent variables. In other words, for 86% of participants, the selected variables correctly identified the participant's answer to the question: "Do you believe you have survived the experience of losing your only child?" For those eight women who were unsure whether they have survived, their responses to the seven independent variables predicted that two belong in the perpetual bereavement group, while six belong in the survival group.

The seven variables included in the discriminant analysis were also used to perform stepwise multiple regression analysis (forward method). Four of the seven variables entered the equation ($p = <.05$), as follows: (1) helpfulness of friends ($R2 = .20$); (2) volunteer activities of participants ($R2 = .09$); (3) amount of time to anticipate child might die ($R2 = .06$); and (4) annual family income ($R2 = .04$). These four independent variables account for a total of 39% of the variance in LABI scores. In other words, 39% of a participant's LABI score may be accounted for by how she answered the questions represented by these four independent variables.

Comparison of Discriminant Group Responses

I used the predicted group membership defined by the discriminant analysis to classify the 80 participants as either remaining perpetually bereaved (n = 18) or as having survived (n = 62). I calculated the frequency of responses to questions on the Participant Questionnaire for these two "predicted" groups and looked for any substantial differences between them. I then performed chi-square analysis to determine statistical significance. Results are shown in Table 1.

The predicted groups from the discriminant analysis (Table 1) and the interviews of mothers with the lowest and highest LABI scores suggest the following profiles of perpetual bereavement and survival:

TABLE 1. Comparison of Responses to Participant Questionnaire by Discriminant Groups

Response to Questionnaire	Perpetual Bereavement (n = 18) Frequency (%)	Survival (n = 62) Frequency (%)	χ^2 (80)
Type of Death:			0.00
Disease or illness	5 (27.8)	17 (27.4)	
Accident	13 (72.2)	45 (72.6)	
Time Between Diagnosis/Accident and Child's Death:			6.53
No warning	9 (50.0)	34 (54.8)	
Hours	4 (22.2)	11 (17.7)	
Days	0 (0)	7 (11.3)	
Weeks	0 (0)	1 (1.6)	
Months	3 (16.7)	2 (3.2)	
Years	2 (11.1)	6 (9.7)	
No response	0 (0)	1 (1.6)	
Time Between Realization Child Might Die and Actual Death:#			3.88
No warning	13 (72.2)	39 (62.9)	
Hours	3 (16.7)	11 (17.7)	
Days	0 (0)	6 (9.7)	
Weeks	1 (5.6)	1 (1.6)	
Months	1 (5.6)	2 (3.2)	
Years	0 (0)	3 (4.8)	
Changed religion after death:			1.15
No	7 (38.9)	33 (53.2)	
Yes	11 (61.1)	29 (46.8)	
Spiritual/religious beliefs helpful:#			3.86
No	6 (33.3)	11 (17.7)	
Both helpful & unhelpful	5 (27.8)	11 (17.7)	
Yes	7 (38.9)	40 (64.5)	
Importance of religion			2.76
Not very important	6 (33.3)	17 (27.4)	
Somewhat important	4 (22.2)	9 (14.5)	
Important	5 (27.8)	13 (21.0)	
Very important	3 (16.7)	23 (37.1)	
Level of grief felt now:			15.96**
Grief dominates life	3 (16.7)	0 (0)	
Feel grief daily	8 (44.4)	24 (38.7)	
Feel grief weekly	3 (16.7)	16 (25.8)	
Feel grief occasionally	3 (16.7)	22 (35.5)	
No longer grieve	1 (5.6)	0 (0)	
Discuss grief with others today:#			25.12**
Never	3 (16.7)	1 (1.6)	
Rarely	8 (44.4)	4 (6.5)	
Occasionally	4 (22.2)	42 (67.7)	
Often	3 (16.7)	15 (24.2)	

Response to Questionnaire	Perpetual Bereavement (n = 18) Frequency (%)	Survival (n = 62) Frequency (%)	χ^2 (80)
Helpfulness of Family:			13.17**
Very unhelpful	6 (33.3)	3 (4.8)	
Unhelpful	4 (22.2)	9 (14.5)	
Somewhat helpful	4 (22.2)	22 (35.5)	
Very helpful	4 (22.2)	28 (45.2)	
Helpfulness of Friends: #			47.89**
Very unhelpful	8 (44.4)	0 (0)	
Unhelpful	6 (33.3)	3 (4.8)	
Somewhat helpful	3 (16.7)	21 (33.9)	
Very helpful	1 (5.6)	38 (61.3)	
Attend Support Group(s):			12.99**
Never attended	3 (16.7)	2 (3.2)	
Once or twice	2 (11.1)	7 (11.3)	
Occasionally	10 (55.6)	16 (25.8)	
Regularly	3 (16.7)	37 (59.7)	
Still Attend Support Group(s):			1.24
No	11 (61.1)	34 (54.8)	
Yes	4 (22.2)	25 (40.3)	
N/A or missing	3 (16.7)	3 (4.8)	
Grief Therapy:			4.19
Never	5 (27.8)	22 (35.5)	
Once or twice	3 (16.7)	11 (17.7)	
Occasionally	6 (33.3)	8 (12.9)	
Regularly	4 (22.2)	21 (33.9)	
Significant losses before child's death:			0.14
Yes	16 (88.9)	53 (85.5)	
No	2 (11.1)	9 (14.5)	
Significant life changes 2 yrs prior:			0.32
No	10 (55.6)	39 (62.9)	
Yes	8 (44.4)	23 (37.1)	
Significant losses after child's death:			5.36*
Yes	18 (100)	47 (75.8)	
No	0 (0)	15 (24.2)	
Learned from motherhood:			0.89
No	1 (5.6)	1 (1.6)	
Yes	17 (94.4)	61 (98.4)	
Current relationships with children			7.80*
No	9 (50.0)	17 (27.4)	
Yes and No	2 (11.1)	1 (1.6)	
Yes	7 (38.9)	44 (71.0)	

TABLE 1 (continued)

Response to Questionnaire	Perpetual Bereavement (n = 18) Frequency (%)	Survival (n = 62) Frequency (%)	X^2 (80)
Marital Status:			11 .49*
Married–to father of child	5 (27.8)	32 (51.6)	
Married–not to father of child	3 (16.7)	13 (21.0)	
Single–divorced	5 (27.8)	14 (22.6)	
Single–never married	2 (11.1)	0 (0)	
Widowed	3 (16.7)	3 (4.8)	
Volunteer Work: #			22.94**
Does not currently volunteer.	14 (77.8)	12 (19.4)	
Volunteered before death, not now	1 (5.6)	2 (3.2)	
Started volunteering after death	2 (11.1)	29 (46.8)	
Volunteered before and after death	1 (5.6)	19 (30.6)	
Employment:			2.62
Not currently employed	2 (11.1)	16 (25.8)	
Started work after death	3 (16.7)	14 (22.6)	
Worked before and after death.	13 (72.2)	32 (51.6)	
Occupation:			7.16
Clerical	6 (33.3)	9 (14.5)	
Service/sales	4 (22.2)	12 (19.4)	
Technical/arts	0 (0)	2 (3.2)	
Professional	2 (11.1)	16 (25.8)	
Managerial	4 (22.2)	7 (11.3)	
Not currently employed	2 (11.1)	16 (25.8)	
Find work meaningful:			0.44
No	4 (22.2)	8 (12.9)	
Yes.	12 (66.7)	38 (61.3)	
No response	2 (11.1)	16 (25.8)	
Education: #			1.13
Less than high school	1 (5.6)	1 (1.6)	
High school graduate	9 (50.0)	29 (46.8)	
College graduate	4 (22.2)	18 (29.0)	
Advanced degree(s)	4 (22.2)	14 (22.6)	
Annual Family Income:#			10.93*
Less than $10,000	1 (5.6)	1 (1.6)	
$10,000 – $24,999	6 (33.3)	4 (6.5)	
$25,000 – $49,999	6 (33.3)	26 (41.9)	
$50,000 – $99,999	4 (22.2)	21 (33.9)	
$100,000 and above	1 (5.6)	10 (16.1)	
Believe survived child's death:			23.03**
No	9 (50.0)	3 (4.8)	
Yes	7 (38.9)	53 (85.5)	
Yes and No	2 (11.1)	6 (9.7)	

#= Discriminating variable used to determine group membership.
* = p < .05
** = p < .01

Profile of Perpetual Bereavement

Those remaining perpetually bereaved continue to experience high levels of grief yet generally they do not discuss their grief with others. They are not actively involved in a grief support group, and they perceive their family and/or friends as unhelpful to them. They do not have significant relationships with other children, and they are not involved in volunteer activities within their community. They may have experienced a significant loss since their child's death. They may have a low standard of living.

The five mothers scoring LOWEST on the LABI experience the loss of their only child as identity disintegration: loss of self, goals, purpose for living, and future. To them, living a new, purposeful life would mean forgetting their child, denying their child's existence, and invalidating their past life as a mother.

> It was my job to be Mommy. I got fired from my job and I don't know why.–Doris

> Sometimes you think, man, is this ever gonna get over with. But then you think, well, you don't want it over with, cause you think if you do, then you'll forget.–Fran

All five of these mothers lack an adequate support system and coping skills. They are hesitant to reach out to others for help and continue to experience recurrent grief, helplessness, mental instability, and physical ailments related to stress.

> I still have periods that I have to take off work, and I have migraines really bad then. . . . I just get really depressed. I get really, really down, and it's hard for me to get back up. . . . I think I hate everybody and everything and just go in (to work) with a chip on my shoulder. Any little thing and I'll fly off the handle. I think it's just mostly anger that he's gone.–Fran

> I feel like a time bomb ready to explode. I don't know from one moment to the next how I'm gonna react or think or do. . . . I'm just totally a different person from it. Brad was my whole life. That was the one thing I wanted was to have a child. . . . I don't feel like I have survived hardly at all since I've lost him. I'm just struggling in the water. I can't envision myself functioning and actually living without him.–Anita

These mothers demonstrate ongoing ambivalence about living, remain angry at God and/or their church and have been unable to incorporate their child's death into a beneficial belief system. They have discovered no purpose for living since their child's death. The mothers' focus is on reviewing aspects of their loss and the effect that unresolved grief is having on their lives.

> Don was my life. He's what I looked forward to in gettin old and him gettin married and having a life and making me a grandmother and havin my house filled with little kids runnin around and there's nothin now–absolutely nothin–and it has–it's made me so angry and it made me so angry at God that this happened. . . . Everything that I had, that I looked forward to in getting old was taken and it's like my mind just stops right there. I can't see any further than that. I can't imagine what else there would be. I want somebody to tell me what I'm spose to be doin.–Ellen

I also found reason to hope that these five women with the lowest LABI scores eventually will be able to heal and reinvest in life. Each had made difficult choices or decisions in the past, indicating the potential for being able to make a future decision to survive the death of their child and live life "alive" again.

Profile of Survival

Grief no longer dominates the lives of the women in the predicted survival group. They are apt to discuss the grief they do feel with others, often at grief support groups. They perceive their family and friends as helpful to them. They are likely to have remained married to their child's father and to have established significant relationships with other children since their child's death. They are also very likely to be involved in some type of volunteer activity within their community. Their family income level may be $50,000 or above per year.

The five mothers scoring HIGHEST on the LABI have experienced the loss of their only child as an identity crisis: loss of part of the self, goals, purpose for living, and future. The child is seen as a separate and distinct personality and the self is seen as possessing unique attributes and strengths.

> I died when he died. Gradually I've birthed a new me. I'm totally different. I have an identity beyond being a mother. . . . I see now that I left Compassionate Friends because I sensed that being a bereaved parent was them–their identity. That's not me. It's a part of who I am and my experience, but it's not the total me.–Gail

These five mothers have made a conscious decision to survive and to reinvest in life. All sought and accepted help from others and learned to use a wide variety of coping skills to deal with their grief and take care of themselves. Nonsupportive family and friends have been replaced with new, understanding others. All continue to experience periodic shadow grief and see bereavement as an evolving, lifelong learning process with some positive benefits.

> You have to make a conscious decision that you will not cling to (your child's) friends–that you will not cling to the old days. You have to go beyond that. . . . I had to reinvent my life. . . . I said, well I've got to keep going if only so Bobby will give me the thumbs up when I get to heaven and say 'good for you Momma, you hung in there and you survived.' I just said, I have to reach out and just keep going. . . . That's basically the way I thought Bobby would want me to be. And it's not that I love him any less, it's just that you have to go on and you have to make a life. You either have to make a life or you have to give up on life and just become a hermit and live with your own pity party. I don't think that's healthy.–Irene

These five women have regained self-control and integrated what they have learned from bereavement into a new identity and a new worldview. Purpose in life is now focused on maintaining a connection with the child and using mothering skills to nurture themselves and others through volunteer activities (such as starting or leading a bereaved parents support group; becoming a hospice volunteer; volunteering in school programs). They see themselves as having become better people.

> After Bobby's death I found compassion for other people that I did not know existed in my personality. I can walk in a room sometimes now and I can zero in on the one person that's in that room that is hurting terribly for whatever reason. It's like a homing device. It has–Bobby's death has made me a much better person. It's made me aware that everyone out there in the entire world belongs to a family. And everybody loves; everybody grieves; everybody hurts; everybody has joy. It's another lesson that God is teaching me in this journey that I'm on to survive the death of my son.–Irene

These five women all learned from prior life crises which may have strengthened their self-esteem. All have acted courageously in confronting their grief by finding or creating opportunities to maintain a connection with their child and their identity as a mother while reinvesting in a purposeful life. All have taken responsibility for their own healing.

Additional Findings

Several other noteworthy (although not statistically significant) findings were drawn from the statistical analysis. While 50% of the predicted perpetual bereavement group shown in Table 1 had no warning between the time of diagnosis or accident and the actual death of their child, 72% of this group said they had no warning the child might die. Likewise, while 55% of the survival group had no warning between the time of diagnosis or accident and the actual death of their child, 63% said they had no warning the child might die. Thus, when the child's death was not immediate as a result of serious illness or accident, such a potential outcome was not anticipated by many mothers. In some cases, the diagnosis given may not have included the possibility of death; in others the mother may not have consciously processed the possibility of her child's dying even when such a possibility was pointed out by doctors. Such was the case for two of the women interviewed:

> Doris—(mother of four year old diagnosed at age two with cerebral palsy): We were never told anything. I mean people live with seizures their whole lives. We knew this was something we might have to deal with the rest of his life, but nobody ever told us it would be fatal.

> Carol—(mother of 15 year old diagnosed at age two with Duschenes muscular dystrophy): It bothers me at all the seminars that I attend and they say, over and over again, when you have a child that is dying it's anticipatory death. Baloney. There's no such thing. Hope and love looks all around. There is no death that's anticipated, nor the same you'd think it'd be when it occurs. And that minimizes my pain and sorrow, and I hope the professionals will stop it. . . . Nothing prepares you. Nothing conditions you for the death of a child. . . . It is not meant to be. And I don't know what they mean, preparation. Maybe you are relieved to see the end of the pain, depending on the situation, but that certainly doesn't—what happens then, what they're thinking is that you miss them less because you had time to prepare and to think. That's untrue.
>
> I will not accept the term acceptance. I feel this way and this is what I say to our [support group] members and when I speak to groups on grief. What do you mean by acceptance? If you mean that I am to accept this unacceptable reality which is against all the laws of nature of burying your child before yourself, I'll say no. If you mean acceptance is letting go of some of the pain associated with the

death, then I will say, ok. However, that isn't the way the term
acceptance is used. So I have to look at things that will help us to
reinvest into life, and that to me is coming to a resolution that my
child always was and always will be a part of my life, and [if] you
allow me to do that, then I can resolve myself to the fact that I will
have to live without him physically the rest of my life. But if you
don't allow him to remain a part of my life, then that's going to put a
wedge in our relationship.

My best friend was my sister-in-law. She's a nurse. We were very
close. But she has pained me so. I've forgiven her, but I can't have a
closeness with her again. . . . She said to me: 'You knew Scott was
going to die from the time you were told he had muscular dystro-
phy.' She says: 'Now put him away and put it aside and get on with
your life.' And she has five healthy children! And she never allowed
me to say his name again.

In some cases hospital staff attempted to force mothers to face the
reality of their child's probable death, resulting in additional trauma:

Gail–(mother of 16 year old who died from head injuries eight days
after a car accident): I would just always say to the neurologists:
What do you need next? What do you need to see next to make you
feel like there's a possibility here? And they'd tell me what they
needed to see next and then I would go tell Andy, this is what they
need to see next. . . . And they just kept being amazed that he was
still alive.

Within that 24-hour period when I first got there, there was a
nurse that came on shift. Actually it was probably sometime Satur-
day or Sunday. And she came into me and she said, 'I need to let you
know that I've heard about you. And I'm not going to participate in
your charades. Your son is going to die. That's a fact. And you might
as well start accepting it.' And I said, 'I need you to know that I'm
going to your supervisor right now. I don't know where she's at. I
don't care if she's here or she's at home. But you are never ever ever
to step foot in my son's room. I'm paying $700 a day for that room. I
have some say-so about who goes in and who doesn't.'

They tried to put me on Valium, which infuriated me. And I again
told them, 'I might seem out of control sometimes. I might seem
hysterical sometimes. I might break down and cry sometimes. Those
are my emotions. I am going to feel them. If you don't like it, then do
your best to stay away from me. Because I'm going to experience
whatever it is I experience. I'm going to be available for this child.'

So they thought I was pretty weird. And I'm sure they thought I was pretty difficult.

The statistical analysis also revealed that 65% of the survival group felt their spiritual or religious beliefs were helpful to them, compared to 39% of the perpetually bereaved group. In addition, 61% of the perpetual bereavement group and 47% of the survival group had changed religions after the death of their child. Fran and Julie provide typical examples:

Fran–(mother of 19 year old who died from head injury four months after a car accident): I had one preacher come up there [to the hospital], and he wanted to pray with me every three hours, and talk to me about now you need to get yourself right with God if you want David to get well. . . . That's not a time for hellfire and brimstone. It's, you know, a time for comfort.

I had one best friend which I've never really forgiven him for it. He told me that if I had been living the kind of life I should have been living, that David wouldn't have died.

There's been times I hated God for taking David away from me. . . . I believe that you pay for what you do or don't do. I don't think God makes your children pay. You know, maybe I'm wrong. I may be totally wrong, but I don't think so.

Julie–(mother of nine year old run over by a drunk driver while standing in the driveway of his home): He [a friend's pastor] opened up the Bible and he says, 'How does it feel to have this link with heaven cause your son's there?' And it was like, um? . . . He read me a passage from the Bible and it said, 'never again to be separated,' that you'll be reunited, never again to be separated. It was like, it hit me like, this is good. I'm here, but this is temporary. . . . Eventually I will be reunited with Stuart. . . . So from this, Pastor M. like opened up my eyes to that, and made it seem like, okey, I have to survive until it's my time. . . . Here I went into Pastor M.'s office . . . and I was in a rage type of a period, but all of a sudden it was like, like just a release, like someone just opened up my head and like just allowed a release of emotion to come out, where it gave me something to hold onto. It gave me something to grasp onto.

CONCLUSIONS

This study supports earlier findings that the death of a child may precipitate a personal transformation in bereaved parents (Cook & Wimberley,

1983; Miles & Crandall, 1986; Wheeler, 1990; Zenoff, 1986). Further, findings imply that a positive life attitude is an indicator of adaptation to this unique form of loss and also may indicate that a personal transformation has occurred. Additional study with a larger sample is necessary to confirm these findings.

Resolving the existential crisis brought about by the death of a child appears to play a crucial part in personal transformation. It seems essential for bereaved parents to find a personally meaningful answer to the question–Where is God when bad things happen? For those of us who have lost an only child, there are many additional questions, for example: What does losing the role of parent mean to my life? How can I honor my child's memory and my past life as a mother and find meaningful ways to reinvest in life again?

Participants who were able to transcend their grief and reconnect with others demonstrated a reordering of priorities in their lives. Having worked through any dissonance in their spiritual beliefs, received adequate support from friends and family, defined the multiple meanings of their relationship with their child and all aspects surrounding the child's death, these women made a conscious decision not to commit suicide but rather to reconnect with others in the world who need empathy and compassion. In return they have regained personal control and experience new meaning and purpose in their lives. The activities they now undertake have become possible not only because their child existed and their role as a mother touched them deeply, but also because their child's death and the pain they have endured in reconciling their grief have created a change in their attitude about life. Surviving the death of their only child has meant a reordering of personal values, responsibility for their own continued healing, and commitment to nurturing themselves and others as they live out their lives as mothers now childless.

REFERENCES

Bevington, K. (1993). *Alive alone.* Van Wert, OH: Alive Alone, Inc.

Cleiren, M. P. H. D. (1993). *Bereavement and adaptation: A comparative study of the aftermath of death.* Washington, DC: Hemisphere Publishing.

Cook, J. A. & Wimberley, D. W. (1983). If I should die before I wake: Religious commitment and adjustment to the death of a child, *Journal of the Scientific Study of Religion,* 22 (3), 222-238.

Ebaugh, H. R. F. (1988). *Becoming an ex: The process of role exit.* Chicago: University of Chicago Press.

Edelstein, L. (1984). *Maternal bereavement: Coping with the unexpected death of a child.* New York: Praeger Publishers.

Giorgi, A. (1975). An application of phenomenological method in psychology. In A. Giorgi, W. Fischer, & E. Murray (Eds.), *Duquesne studies in phenomenological psychology.* (Vol 2, pp. 82-103). Pittsburgh: Duquesne University Press.

Hycner, R. H. (1985). Some guidelines for the phenomenological analysis of interview data, *Human Studies,* 8 (3), 279-303.

Knapp, R. J. (1986). *Beyond endurance: When a child dies.* New York: Schocken Books.

Miles, M. S. & Crandall, E. K. B. (1986). The search for meaning and its potential for affecting growth in bereaved parents. In R. H. Moos (Ed.), *Coping with life crises: An integrated approach,* (pp. 235-243). New York: Plenum Press. (Original work published 1983).

Osterweis, M., Solomon, F., & Green, M. (Eds). (1984). *Bereavement: Reactions, consequences, and care.* Committee for the Study of Health Consequences of the Stress of Bereavement, Institute of Medicine, Washington, DC: National Academy Press.

Rando, T. A. (1986). Parental bereavement: An exception to the general conceptualizations of mourning. In T. A. Rando (Ed.), *Parental loss of a child,* (pp. 45-58). Champaign, IL: Research Press.

Reker, G. T. & Peacock, E. J. (1981). The Life Attitude Profile (LAP): A multidimensional instrument for assessing attitudes toward life. *Canadian Journal of Behavioral Science,* 13, 264-273.

Reker, G. T. (1992). *Manual for the Life Attitude Profile-Revised.* Peterborough, Ontario, Canada: Student Psychologists Press.

Reker, G. T. & Wong, T. P. (1984). Psychological and physical well-being in the elderly: The Perceived Well-Being Scale (PWB)." *Canadian Journal on Aging,* 3 (1), 23-32.

Sanders, C. M. (1979-1980). A comparison of adult bereavement in the death of a spouse, child, and parent, *Omega,* 10, 303-322.

Sanders, C. M. (1989). *Grief: The mourning after–dealing with adult bereavement.* New York: John Wiley & Sons.

Wheeler, I. P. (1990). The role of meaning and purpose in life in parental bereavement. *Dissertation Abstracts International,* 52/04-B, 2319. (University Microfilms No. 91-17334).

Zenoff, N. R. (1986). *The mother's experience after the sudden death of a child: Personal and transpersonal perspectives.* Doctoral dissertation, Institute of Transpersonal Psychology, Menlo Park, CA. (University Microfilms No. LD01052).

Grief and AIDS:
Surviving Catastrophic Multiple Loss

Gail Bigelow
Jeremy Hollinger

SUMMARY. This article explores the issues of grief brought about by the AIDS epidemic. As people affected by the epidemic experience multiple deaths in both their personal and professional lives, the parallel epidemic of grief is reaching crisis proportions. Traditional grief responses are compared with multiple loss grief and appropriate clinical interventions are explored. The phenomena of trauma, survivor guilt, Post-Traumatic Stress Disorder and other historic examples of multiple loss (holocausts) are examined. The existential questions of how to hold hope as we live in an "abyss of trauma, death and grief" concludes this article. *[Article copies available for a fee from The Haworth Document Delivery Service: 1-800-342-9678. E-mail address: getinfo@haworth.com]*

The grief that we feel when one person after another dies, without time for us to recover, defies our traditional understanding of bereavement. The

---

Gail Bigelow, LCSW, holds a Master of Social Welfare and is a Licensed Clinical Social Worker. She is currently the Bereavement Coordinator, Visiting Nurses and Hospice of San Francisco. Jeremy Hollinger, MFCC, holds a Master of Counseling Psychology and is currently a Licensed Marriage, Family and Child Counselor and Assistant Bereavement Coordinator, Visiting Nurses and Hospice of San Francisco.

Address correspondence to: Gail Bigelow, LCSW, Bereavement Coordinator, Visiting Nurses and Hospice of San Francisco, 3360 Geary Boulevard, San Francisco, CA 94118.

[Haworth co-indexing entry note]: "Grief and AIDS: Surviving Catastrophic Multiple Loss." Bigelow, Gail and Jeremy Hollinger. Co-published simultaneously in *The Hospice Journal* (The Haworth Press, Inc.) Vol. 11, No. 4, 1996, pp. 83-96; and: *Bereavement: Client Adaptation and Hospice Services* (ed: Donna Lind Infeld, and Nadine Reimer Penner) The Haworth Press, Inc., 1996, pp. 83-96. Single or multiple copies of this article are available for a fee from The Haworth Document Delivery Service [1-800-342-9678, 9:00 a.m. - 5:00 p.m. (EST). E-mail address: getinfo@haworth.com].

authors of this article coordinate the Bereavement Program of a large urban hospice in which 60% of the patients die of AIDS. The survivors, facing AIDS related loss, are usually grieving more than one loved one, in fact often dozens or even hundreds. This experience of mourning resembles what has been described by victims of war and natural disaster.

In searching for a language and framework to help our clients, our co-workers and ourselves, we, the authors, have turned to the work that has been done with trauma survivors to enhance our understanding of the nature of this extraordinary grief. Many of our clients report that this way of understanding what they are going through brings some relief, that at least it helps them name the experience.

> In the midst of winter
> I finally learned
> there is in me
> an invincible summer
>
> –Camus (1954)

To begin with, we turn to the work of leading investigators in the field of grief and loss: Eric Lindemann (1944), Elizabeth Kübler-Ross (1969), John Bowlby (1980), Colin Murray Parkes (1972), Therese Rando (1984), and J. William Worden (1991), to name a few. Each of these scholars describes the experience of bereavement in their own terms, agreeing on some basic tenets. They concur that grief is a normal response to the loss of someone to whom you are attached; that it affects you physically, emotionally, cognitively, behaviorally and spiritually; and that everyone grieves uniquely. In general, after the death of a loved one, we go through the process of (1) shock/numbness, (2) suffering/disorganization, (3) recovery/adjustment. We have found Worden's (1991) conceptualization of the four tasks of grief to be especially helpful in our work with clients. Diagram 1 is a visual depiction of his concepts.

Task A: To accept the reality of the loss.

Task B: To work through the pain of the grief.

Task C: To adjust to an environment in which the deceased is missing.

Task D: To emotionally relocate the deceased and move on with life.

Many cultures around the world recognize grief and ritualize mourning much more than is common in the U.S. Beyond the funeral and the official

DIAGRAM 1

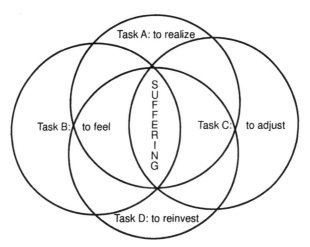

three days of bereavement leave from work, there is very little social validation that the survivor is adjusting to what may be a radically life changing event. The hospice movement and the growth of bereavement support services have made a dent in the social isolation many grievers feel, but we have far to go. One of our clients participates in drop-in bereavement support groups in "chat rooms" on line!

AIDS AND BEREAVEMENT

When normal grief is stigmatized, how much more so is AIDS-related grief, which follows the HIV epidemic like a shadow. Because the epidemic has primarily affected the gay men's community and injection drug users, some conservative politicians have successfully pandered to people's homophobia, racism and fear by casting this illness as God's punishment.

> AIDS is God's way of punishing those who break
> the laws of nature and the laws of moral decency . . .
> The Scripture is clear: we do reap it in our flesh when
> we violate the laws of God.

> –Jerry Falwell, *Oakland Tribune*, July 13, 1983

The consequent shame that many people feel when grieving an AIDS-related loss severely complicates the grief: the mother who returned to

Texas from San Francisco after caring for her son who died of AIDS asked that we not mail her anything because she told everyone he died of cancer; the gay man who could not tell anyone at work about his partner's death because of his fear of being fired if they knew he was gay; the roommate who hid his friend's illness from the landlord for fear of being evicted; the little girl who was terrified that her teachers or classmates at her parochial school might find out that her mother was dying of AIDS. This inability to speak about the great pain of grief cuts like a knife and inhibits recovery.

In addition to the cruelty of society, we are coping with the cruelty of this disease. Most of the people we are grieving are young, in their 20s, 30s and 40s. Many of us grieving can say that some of the kindest, funniest, brightest, most beautiful, most warm-hearted people we have known have died of this illness. They are parents of young children, people still in the early years of contributing their gifts to society, people of courage. People coping with AIDS-related loss are often grieving their peers and the loss of their community.

In the gay communities and drug using communities, alternative family and support structures have sprung up–families of choice. Often, these relations are not recognized or accepted by the family of origin or other people in positions of authority. Parents and siblings may take over a patient's care at the very end of his life, refusing to allow the partner, who provided the long term care, any decision-making power. They may take all of the possessions at the time of death and may blame the partner for their family member's death. Further, few workplaces give financial benefits to non-traditional partners.

The bereaved are often HIV positive themselves, vulnerable to the same fate. They may be coping with their own physical status and facing their own mortality while they are grieving the loss of their dear ones, and perhaps feel exhausted from months of providing primary care. The physical symptoms of grief and HIV can exacerbate and look like each other, as in the following examples:

AIDS Symptoms	Grief Symptoms
pneumonia	tightness in the chest
wasting	weight loss
no energy	fatigue
dementia	difficulty concentrating

This can be overwhelmingly frightening, and accentuates the need for HIV positive bereaved individuals to be under the care of AIDS-competent medical doctors.

We're all going to go crazy, living the epidemic every
minute, while the rest of the world goes on out there . . .
as if nothing is happening . . . not knowing what it's like . . .
we're living through war, but where they're living it's
peacetime, and we're all in the same country.

–Larry Kramer, *The Normal Heart* (1985)

MULTIPLE LOSS

Running parallel to the AIDS epidemic is the secondary epidemic of
grief. What is it like for people who are grieving many losses at the same
time due to AIDS? They cannot complete one task of grief before losing
another loved one. Try to understand this experience by imagining yourself in the center of concentric circles, each one a layer of loss. Perhaps
you are HIV positive yourself, and you are grieving the loss of your own
health. You may be feeling nauseous, exhausted or in pain. You may have
lost your job and your financial security. One circle out, perhaps your
lover and daily support person has died and you are feeling all that comes
with widowhood. Perhaps your dearest friends have died, one after the
other, and most, or all, who have known you over the years and shared
your memories are now gone. Your family of choice is radically altered,
perhaps vanished.

Going a layer further out, your world has changed. Many of your
acquaintances, co-workers, clients, professionals whom you do business
with have died. The friendly face at the grocery store or the bank is gone.
On another further layer, your culture, your community identity, your
feelings of having a future are no longer there.

This grief is frightening, tiring, and overwhelming. It resembles the
experience of many elderly people, forcing people in their early and mid-
life to face the developmental tasks most people confront in their 60s, 70s
and 80s. Instead of focusing on finding identity, contributing through
work, forging relationships and a family, they grapple with death and the
meaning of life. This kind of grief may look less and less like the more
traditional acute grief we are familiar with. It begins to pervade all of life
and become a generalized state of being. It can be like the smog of urban
areas–always present, often unseen, and doing its hidden damage. We
become so immersed in it, we cease to notice it any more.

TRAUMA

The work "trauma" comes from the Greek root meaning "to wound."
While any loss or death may prove traumatic, some losses are of such

magnitude as to require further study. Three other man-made holocausts share similar characteristics with the AIDS epidemic which many also consider a holocaust. Like the AIDS epidemic, the magnitude of the Jewish holocaust, the nuclear holocaust in Japan, and the Cambodian holocaust stand out. Five features are unique to each of these four:

1. The total life experience is disrupted. Unlike a single stressful event that takes place against a backdrop of normal psychological and social functioning, these conditions replace the total fabric of normal life with a surrealistic existence, unanchored in familiar elements of reality.
2. The new environment is extremely hostile, threatening, and dangerous.
3. Opportunities to remove or act upon the stressor environment are severely limited.
4. There is no predictable end to the experience.
5. The pain and suffering associated with the experience appear to be meaningless and without rational explanation. (Kahana, 1988, p. 59)

These five factors also characterize the lives of clients who are grieving the loss of their entire world of relationships. The perception that, inevitably, everyone will die, there is no way out, and that the world is no longer safe is reflected in the following statements of two different members of our Multiple Loss Bereavement Group:

> It does seem like everyone is dying. Every dick is a loaded gun. I walk down Castro Street, and whereas before there were many familiar faces, today I don't know anyone. In the seventies, I knew all the shop keepers on the Castro. Today, they are all dead and strangers have taken their place. I feel that all we had worked to create is disappearing.

> I was in Vietnam and saw many people die there. When out on patrol, we always sent a point man out first to see if he'd draw enemy fire. His presence protected the rest of us. In the epidemic, I feel like our point man is being knocked out and my cover is gone. Our protection was in our numbers, and now they are gone. And I am exposed. I am no longer protected. Life is not safe.

In addition, the DSM IV's description of Post-Traumatic Stress Disorder rings true (keeping in mind that the multiple loss experience is ongoing, not "post"):

> Symptoms that follow a psychologically distressing event that is outside the range of normal human experience and would be dis-

tressing to anyone and produce fear, terror, and helplessness. . . . The person has been exposed to a traumatic even in which both of the following were present:

1. The person experienced, witnessed or was confronted with an event or events that involved actual or threatened death or serious injury, or a threat to the physical integrity of self or others.
2. The person's response involved intense fear, helplessness or horror.

Conway (1991), in an interview at the National Center for Post-Traumatic Stress Disorder, gives this description of PTSD:

> PTSD is a psychic injury, just like any other injury to the body. If you lie in the sun, you will tan. But if you stay too long, you'll burn. The mind is like the skin, except it responds to experience. Instead of tanning, the mind has emotional reactions and makes decisions. If the experience heats up enough, the mind will burn. That burn is PTSD. (p. 6)

Multiple loss grief is not just a personal experience of overwhelming trauma, but also a communal experience with as dramatic an impact upon the communities affected as that of the citizens of Buffalo Creek when the community dam broke and destroyed the lives of thousands (Erickson, 1976).

The survivors of the Buffalo Creek disaster suffered both individual and collective traumas, the latter being reflected in their loss of communality . . . the survivors experienced demoralization, disorientation, and loss of connection. Stripped of the support they had received from their community, they became apathetic and seemed to have forgotten how to care for one another (p. 302).

> There is no shame
> in avoiding elephants.

> –Vietnamese Proverb, *A Rumor of Angels*
> In Perry and Perry (1989)

NUMBING AND FLOODING

We have found that many of our clients (and our co-workers and ourselves) cope with the intense emotion and anxiety of the "unbearable" loss they are experiencing with two very important skills: numbing and flooding (see Diagram 2). Numbing refers to our ability to turn off our emotions, to avoid painful thoughts and images, to deny the full impact of our grief. It may feel like depression, going through the motions, wooden, moving under water, feeling distant from people and events. This capacity allows us to process the pain in small doses, to reduce our anxiety while we gradually come to terms with the reality of losing so many loved ones so quickly. However, all of us who have used this skill for a long time know that feeling numb is very far from feeling good. In fact, it can lead to hopelessness, fatigue, and suicidal feelings.

We have found that a key therapeutic intervention is assisting clients in gaining some *control* in moving between the states of numbing and flooding. By moving between these states, we can process the trauma over time and find some hope, peace and inner strength again. It may be helpful to encourage clients to learn to avoid by changing the furniture, putting away

DIAGRAM 2. Our Emotional Process: The Emotional Reaction to Trauma

Emotional Pendulum

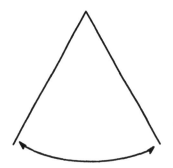

Flooding of emotion	Numbness
Hyperarousal, edginess	Depression
Increased fear	Denial
Difficulty concentrating	Attempts to avoid painful thoughts, images and feelings
Sleep disturbance	
Attempts to process and integrate the pain	Feeling nothing
	Going through the motions
Easily tearful	Detachment from people and events

reminders of their grief, traveling different routes so as not to pass certain places. It is very important for them to steer away from the desire to anesthetize themselves with drugs, alcohol, unsafe sex and other self destructive behaviors, and instead to identify soothing, healthy, distracting activities to turn to when they want to stop their thoughts and feelings. Social support is key. It helps to be able to call up a friend and go do something. This is another great value of bereavement support groups–the forming of new and trusting friendships. The support group can become the safe place to learn the skill of opening up and then closing down.

The flooding side of this emotional pendulum may be experienced as hyperarousal, edginess, fear, difficulty concentrating, sleep disturbance and tearfulness. Again, staying in this state is not a good way to live. Clients learn to open up to the pain and anxiety as a key to processing their changing life situation. Gaining some control over their feelings by letting themselves go into emotion in tolerable doses can be a great comfort. For clients to "tell their story" to others who listen with compassion and understanding in a weekly counseling session or support group is one way of taking charge and "deciding to flood."

Many people are afraid that if they start to emote, they will never finish. As one client said, "I think I will die if I experience these feelings . . . they are so much bigger than I am." The very experience of attending a multiple loss bereavement support group can allow clients to experience opening up and closing down as the group comes to an end each week. Besides bereavement counseling, they may identify safe ways of flooding such as having a special "altar" at home where they put pictures and other mementos (which by its nature also provides a container for all the losses), creating a ritual (lighting a candle or talking to those who have died) at a set time, listening to music or watching a movie that will make them cry, or screaming on the beach. Again, assisting clients in gaining some control over when they flood and when they turn numb, and framing both as positive (necessary) adaptive skills, greatly increases their feelings of power in the midst of overwhelming trauma that can feel so out of control.

We should never underestimate the empowering nature of a support group. Many clients feel they are the only ones having these "fears of feelings," and the experience of having lost all that is most valuable in their life. They report that friends do not want to hear about their grief, and others outside the community do no understand it. The ritual of gathering in a support group to tell stories gives the first sense that they do have some control over the epidemic, even if it is only the formation of their own attitudes and strategies for survival. In the safety of others who know the same experience, many find their feelings are not the Pandora's Box they had feared.

SURVIVOR GUILT

Another complicating emotion for many bereaved is survivor guilt, especially if they are HIV negative. They have lived the same way as many of their friends who have died, yet they have escaped this disease. They ask, "Why not me?" Benefitting from the irrational striking down of some, but not others, can be immobilizing. At the same time, living with so much loss may not feel like such a stroke of luck. Many are overcome with despair, hopelessness and anxiety. They do not feel they have a future worth living for, and develop a desire to die. In many places, prevention and support services for HIV negative people are growing in recognition of the emotional weight they are carrying. It is vital that this survivor guilt be named as a normal part of grief, and that people be encouraged to live. We all need the message that it is a good and worthwhile thing to take care of ourselves. When taking care of ourselves may require time out from personal or professional care giving duties, guilt can make it very difficult to say no to the many urgent needs of friends and clients.

As service providers in the HIV epidemic, we and our co-workers are not immune from survivor guilt and also the need to swing between flooding and numbing. Betty Carmack, professor from the School of Nursing at the University of San Francisco, has developed a chart that describes the functional and dysfunctional sides of both states, which she names engagement and detachment. Diagram 3 is a visual depiction of her concepts. Perhaps we can recognize ourselves being in each of these four squares on different days. Hopefully, we usually stay on the functional side of the grid moving between functional engagement and functional detachment. It seems an essential skill to be able to detach and "have a life outside of AIDS" in order to be able to do this kind of work for more than a short time.

SHATTERED ASSUMPTIONS

Sorrow makes us all children again—
destroys all differences in intellect. The
wisest know nothing.

–Ralph Waldo Emerson (1842)

DIAGRAM 3

CARING	BURNOUT
FUNCTIONAL ENGAGEMENT ○ Self fulfilled by supporting other while protecting against overinvolvement ○ Made a difference ○ Emotional involvement manageable	DYSFUNCTIONAL ENGAGEMENT ○ Overinvolved ○ Overwhelmed ○ Saturated ○ Burned out ○ Cannot regulate giving
FUNCTIONAL DETACHMENT ○ More detached—feels OK to protect self from emotional pain ○ Time off—"Convalescence" ○ "Turns off" one's mind ○ "A life outside of AIDS"	DYSFUNCTIONAL DETACHMENT ○ Numbness ○ Uninvolved ○ Feels it makes no difference in another's life ○ Dissatisfied with this degree of detachment ○ Isolated ○ Increased alcohol/drugs ○ Won't make friends with PWHIV or PWA

Ronnie Janoff-Bulman's work with trauma survivors is particularly enlightening to our understanding of multiple loss. She outlines three assumptions that most of us hold if we have had a reasonably positive life experience (1992):

1. The world is benevolent.
    a. People are basically good and kind.
    b. Events that happen to me are more often positive than negative.
2. The world is meaningful.
    a. There is a relationship between a person and what happens to him/her: good things happen to good people.
    b. We can control what happens to us through our behavior.
    c. Events are orderly and understandable.
3. I am worthy.
    a. I am good, decent and moral.
    b. I deserve credit for the positive things that happen to me.
    c. I control what happens to me.

Janoff-Bulman found that most of us selectively remember successes over failures, and that we tend to be unrealistically optimistic, discounting the possible negative outcomes and risk factors in our environments. This adaptive denial works to our advantage by helping us feel positive emotions, act more positively towards others and therefore increase positive outcomes in our lives. However, these foundations of trust fall apart when something terrible happens. Instead of being able to change slowly over time, we are faced with an abrupt disruption of our inner security.

These assumptions seem matched to the U.S. culture: this is "the land of opportunity." The individual is responsible for what happens to him or her, if you work hard you will be successful. Suffering is stigmatized in our culture–if something bad happens to you, you must have deserved it. This is in contrast to Buddhist culture, for instance, which understands suffering as an integral and inevitable part of life. Of course, if we have had generally negative life experiences from the time of our childhood, we probably hold to opposite assumptions about our worth and the world's benevolence. We may still view the world as meaningful (I am bad, therefore bad things happen to me). Additional trauma probably just entrenches us in our fear and isolation.

Researchers have found that victims of human-induced trauma, such as rape, are mainly shaken in their beliefs about their own worth and others' goodness. Natural disasters, on the other hand, shatter the "order and meaning" of the victim's world. Horrible things can happen out of the blue.

HIV and multiple loss, in a sense, are both. An epidemic is an "act of God," outside of human control. However, people with HIV and those grieving AIDS-related loss must also face the cruelty of other people's prejudice, including, perhaps, their own internalized homophobia and/or racism.

> Everything can be taken from a man
> but one thing: the last of the human
> freedoms–to choose one's attitude . . .
> to choose one's own way.
>
> –Victor Frankl (1959)

Our main task in recovering from a trauma is to reinterpret it in such a way that it is integrated into a more complex and sophisticated view of the world that again affirms the possibility of goodness in ourselves and others. We have probably all been drawn to people who have "been through a lot," yet, instead of their pain resulting in bitterness, they are able to live their lives with increased wisdom, humor and compassion. It is certainly true that any tragedy can give us the gift of empathy with others going through a similar hardship.

One of the ways we try to come to terms with a trauma is to compare our situation to something worse . . . "Thank God I'm still alive." On a deeper level, we struggle to find meaning in the pain. Victor Frankl's courage and insight in the concentration camp can guide us. He was able to see that no outward cruelty could break his inner integrity—that he could triumph above all that was done to him (Frankl, 1959). Likewise, the AIDS epidemic puts many of the deepest spiritual questions before those who are affected: Who am I? What is the meaning of my life? Do I die when my body dies? All of the great spiritual traditions pose this contemplation of death as a key practice toward a higher state of consciousness. Many are attracted to doing hospice work for the very reason that it leads us to the edge of this mystery that connects us all. It is a profound state to be able to hold the anguish brought about by the epidemic and at the same time feel peace and respect for each person who is dying, recognizing that for them, this is their particular death and that there is nothing wrong with it.

Another way to find meaning in the trauma is to take action. This may be action for yourself, such as joining a support group, taking care of your own health, creating something (art, music, dance, poetry), participating in ritual (the Names Quilt, for example), saying no to a request for more care giving. Or it may be more outward oriented action: joining a political group to pressure Congress for more AIDS funding, joining a speakers bureau to talk to youth about safe sex, contributing money to AIDS services. Even small acts can counter the powerless feeling that arises from the hugeness of the epidemic. As one client said in our Coping with Multiple Loss support group, "If I can't see the light at the end of the tunnel, I'll string the lights along the way." Another client defined hope as believing a person can make a difference. Victor Frankl quotes Nietzsche's words, "He who has a why to live for can bear with almost any how." In Frankl's experience of surviving a Nazi concentration camp, any suffering can be borne which the individual could give meaning to (Frankl, 1959, p. 97). For each person, this meaning is unique.

Without doubt, this loss is extraordinary and hope can be the most elusive of feelings. Even to mention the word "hope" in our Multiple Loss groups is to invite a hostile reaction. This reaction presents us with the ultimate questions the survivors face: Can we find hope, tenderness, and peace in our hearts int he midst of such a holocaust? Is there a future? Will there be a community for me? Community is key to the question of surviving with hope. While I alone may feel overwhelmed, as part of a community seeking to make some sense of our experience, I can go on. We turn for guidance to the words of Lu Xun, a Chinese poet who lived from 1881 to 1936.

Hope can be neither affirmed or denies.
Hope is like a path in the countryside;
originally there was no path.
Yet, as people walk all the time in the same spot,
a way appears.

(in Bidgood, 1992)

REFERENCES

American Psychiatric Association. (1994). *Diagnostic and statistical manual of mental disorders* (Fourth Edition). Washington, D.C.: Author.

Bowlby, J. (1980). *Attachment and loss: Loss, sadness and depression.* (Vol. lll). New York: Basic Books.

Camus, A. (1954). *L'ETE,* Paris: Gallimard.

Carmack, B. (1992). *Balancing engagement/detachment in aids-related multiple loss.* IMAGE: Journal of Nursing Scholarship, Vol. 24, 1, 9-14.

Conway, C. (1991). *Then-now. The Stanford Medicine.* 8(4), 4-8.

Emerson, RW. (1960). *Journals.* Vol. 8: entry for 30 Jan. 1842.

Erickson, K. (1976). *Loss of community at buffalo creek.* American Journal of Psychiatry. 133, 302-305.

Frankl, V. (1959). *Man's search for meaning.* New York: Washington Square Press.

Janoff-Bulman, R. (1992). *Shattered assumptions.* New York: Free Press.

Kahanea, E.; Kahana, B.; Harel, Z.; & Rosner, T. (1988). Coping with extreme trauma. In J. Wilson, Z. Harel, B. Kahana, (Eds.). *Human adaption to extreme stress.* (pp. 55-80). New York: Plenum Press.

Kramer, L. (1985). *The normal heart.* New York City: New American Library.

Kübler-Ross, E. (1969). *On death and dying.* New York: Macmillan.

Lindeman, E. (1944). Symptomology and management of acute grief. *American Journal of Psychiatry, 101,* 141-148.

Parkes, C.M. (1972). *Bereavement: Studies of grief in adult life.* New York: International Universities Press.

Perry, G., & Perry, J., (eds.) (1989). *A rumor of angels.* New York: Ballantine Books.

Rando, T.A. (1984). *Grief, dying and death: Clinical interventions for caregivers.* Champaign, Illinois: Research Press.

Randolph, E. (1983). *Falwell calls on U.S. to curb aids spread.* Oakland: Oakland Tribune.

Worden, J.W. (1991). *Grief counseling and grief therapy.* (Second Edition). New York: Springer.

Xun, Lu. In Bidgood, R. (1992). Coping with the trauma of aids losses. In Land, H., (ed.) *AIDS: a complete guide to psychosocial interventions.* Milwaukee: Family Services of America, Inc.

Index

HIV negative support groups
and, 92
of service providers, 92
trauma and, 87
features of, 88
holocaust similarities and, 88
PTSD similarities to, 88-89
Grief, pathological grief reactions
assessment and, 2

Hospice of Louisville,
interdisciplinary
bereavement team of. *See*
Interdisciplinary
bereavement team

Interdisciplinary bereavement team
benefits of, 21-23
lay volunteer benefits, 22-23
program accountability, 22
support to personnel, 22
"team" spirit, 22
trust levels, 22
wholistic approach to bereaved
families, 22
willingness to take
responsibility, 22
composition of, 19-20
educational or support group
issues and, 19
hospice care interdisciplinary
team and, 15-16
"musicare" program and, 23
program process of
confidentiality, 20
initial case presentation
genogram, 20-21
update case presentations, 21
purpose of
closure after discharge, 18
complicated bereavement case
consultation, 18-19
discussion and debate forum,
18

healthy loss accommodation,
18
limited resources consultation,
19
maintenance of boundaries, 18
referrals when needed, 18
rationale of
alternate perspectives benefit
and, 18
consistency of interventions
and, 17
continuum of need and, 16
counseling vs. therapy concept
and, 17
organization mission and value
and, 16
personnel isolation reduction
and, 18
reasonableness and
appropriateness and, 17
referral for extensive needs
and, 17
replication of model of
community outreach and, 23
counseling/therapy
professionals recruitment
and, 23
simplicity of creation, 23-24
summary regarding, 15-16

Japanese nuclear holocaust trauma,
88
Jewish holocaust trauma, 88,94,95

Kramer, Larry, 87

LABI. *See* Life Attitude Balance
Index
LAP-R (Life Attitude
Profile-Revised), 68-69
death acceptance, 69
existential vacuum, 69

Printed and bound by CPI Group (UK) Ltd, Croydon, CR0 4YY

17/10/2024

01775686-0008